CW00506204

THE POWER TO MOVE FOR SUCCESS

How To Walk Your Talk And Get Exactly What You Want From Life

MARTIN BOOTHE

"Many people don't have a deep connection with their mind, body and spirit. That's the reason they ultimately end up failing in life or becoming a success but still feeling empty and unfulfilled. This book will change all that with its simple messages and proven life, energy and movement success systems."
- Reg Athwal,
International Speaker, Human Potential Expert, and co-Author of
#1 bestseller "Wake up ... Live The Life You Love" series

Published by Sparkwave
First Published 2004

The Power To Move For Success

ISBN 0-9546805-1-0

Copyright © Martin Boothe, 2004

The right of Martin Boothe to be identified as the author of this work has been asserted by him in accordance with the *Copyright, Designs and Patent Act 1988.*

All rights reserved. No part of this book may be reproduced or utilized in any form or by any means, electronic or mechanical, including photocopying, recording or by any information storage and retrieval system, without permission in writing from the Publisher.

Design and illustrations by Richie Amiel of Rigami Design

Printed by Booksurge

You can contact Martin Boothe via moveforsuccess@aol.com

ABOUT THE AUTHOR

Martin Boothe is a coach, a personal trainer, a dance and movement teacher and a choreographer.

He has studied and acquired qualifications in the fields of dance, movement, coaching, counselling, health, fitness and sports psychology. He therefore has a deep and profound understanding of the capacity that everyone has to improve his or her life situation through the use of physiology and psychology.

He delivers workshops and seminars, coaches, teaches and choreographs for thousands of people from all walks of life from around the world.

He was dance and fitness teacher for Andrew Lloyd Webber's hit musical *'Starlight Express'* in Germany for over six years. He is the co-founder of the Responsible Men's Club and creator of the musical *'The Vital Fire'*.

He has a great passion for pursuing excellence in all areas of life, be they physical, emotional, financial or spiritual. He is enthusiastic about creating positive energy that improves the quality of people's lives.

His philosophy is to work with emotion, co-ordination, rhythm, energy, agility and health to really become, live and enjoy what you want in life. It's about getting in touch with the power and the energy of the human body. It's time not to just think about being successful, but to actively be successful. Success not as society might define it, but success as you define it. It's about living your truth and honouring and getting the life you want to live.

"To continue striving to be a better person *and* being all that you can be is a drive from the human spirit. Honouring your mind, body and soul can only be healing in the deepest sense. It is the greatest gift to yourself and the world to live a true and passionate experience."
- Martin Boothe

"Don't think; feel.
It's like a finger pointing to the moon.
Don't concentrate on the finger,
Or you will miss out on all the heavenly glory."
- Bruce Lee in 'Enter the Dragon'

CONTENTS

FOREWORD

At the time of writing, it is coming up to a year that I have known of Martin Boothe's existence on God's green Earth. We met through a mutual friend who had the foresight to know that we must connect, as we would have a lot to talk about.

Our first and only meeting was spent in a café in London talking about what it would be like to write a book. I had just returned from a book seminar in Los Angels teaching the mechanics of how to write, market and promote books so I was filled with fresh information that I was keen to share with anyone that would listen. While we spoke Martin had a look in his eye that he meant business – he had a story to tell, something to share and he felt duty bound to do it.

Over the next eight or so months we communicated via email once in a while. Martin kept me up to date with the progress of his book, until in Jan 2004 I received an e-mail saying, and I quote, *"My book is in its final stages, and will be out hopefully in a few weeks from now."* The timing of this was amazing, as my book was due out around the same time. Less than twelve months previously the book you're now holding, the book you're now reading was nothing more than a concept that started inside of Martin's head. This book was an idea floating on the aroma of freshly ground coffee. Some people have great ideas and thoughts that stay just that, whilst other people have great ideas and thoughts that then become a reality.

Martin belongs in the latter category: he is a 'mover' in every sense of the word.

The techniques shared in this book work – the proof is in the pudding as they say. Martin walks his talk in every way, otherwise this book would still be in his head and you would have to be telepathic in order to read it.

I urge you not just to read this book, as that alone won't change your life. There is not a book on the face of the planet that will change your life just by reading it. You need to act. You need to 'move', much like Martin moved by getting his practices and beliefs into print.

Enjoy.

Peace and love,

Steve Rock
Author of *'Failing Your Way To Success'* and co-author of *'The Inspirational Poet'*.

ACKNOWLEDGEMENTS

The most endearing heartfelt gratitude and thanks to so many people that have been a part of my unique journey and discoveries.

To my wonderful family for being a part of the moulding and creation of the man to write this book.

To Team 5, Hawaii 2001, for sharing a special and enriching learning time together. My dear friend Richie Amiel for his illustrations, friendship, kindness and talents. My main man Lindsay "Linds" who keeps me inspired with his strength, determination, fitness and laughter. Tony Robbins for being a great role model of excellence. Heike Senger for being a passionate beautiful loving soul and gift to my life. Susanne Duesberg for the deep soul connection, her guidance, passion and love, a true beacon of strength and honour to life. The Starlight crew for allowing me to grow, learn and shine. Chris Walsh for her kindness, love and support. Individual Fight Concepts Mallepree brothers, for stretching me to greater heights of achievement. Sue Ellen Shook, a completely gifted soul to whom my connection and friendship transcends the human experience. Tommie, Clive, Kelvin, Ray and Nicky who supported me in the freeing experience of dance. Trevor Hodge for sharing so many memorable moments on stage together. Dwight Toppin for being a beautiful spirit and dear friend.

All these people have been a part of creating the cocktail of the making of me and I honour the hours, days, months and years spent with them.

To all the lives I have touched and moved and to those who have moved me over the years by allowing me to be part of their experience.

PREFACE

I feel truly blessed and I want to acknowledge my appreciation and gratitude for my own body, as well as for the many people who have moved and inspired me through the expression of who they are and the use of their talents, skills and bodies in the form of music, dance, design, art and emotion. They have all been a part of my great journey through life, and have inspired me to put pen to paper.

I've been very fortunate to work alongside some great people over the years such as Madonna, Jennifer Rush, Lenny Henry, Andrew Lloyd Webber, George Takei - who we've known and loved as Sulu on *Star Trek* – as well as learning from some masterful teachers over the years. They have all played a powerful part in my life.

This experience has allowed me to move, inspire and entertain millions of people all over the world. I have been fortunate to be able to do this by using my own physical ability and through being able to express myself emotionally and by learning, growing and achieving through movement.

Because of this, I became aware of how much I've grown emotionally and how much I have been able to transfer that emotion onto others through the expression of myself through my body.

I have also come to realize that my successes in life truly lay in the way I used my body. When I've managed it successfully I've enjoyed success. In this book I want to share with you what I have learned so that you can also enjoy the rich rewards that come to you when you use your body successfully. My aim is simple: I want to demonstrate how you too can *move for success*.

This is about getting in touch with the power and energy of the human body so that you have the power to gain an edge in life, business, health, wealth and relationships. This is about how to master unique qualities of your physiology, so that it always serves you and gives you the power to keep going when others fall.

This book will help you to:

- have more energy
- lose weight in a healthy and powerful way
- suffer fewer illnesses
- achieve better results in business and in your communications
- have more staying power
- have more focus in business
- enjoy more productive hours in the day
- achieve real connection in your close relationships and with others
- achieve more and longer-lasting success

IT'S TIME TO FINALLY GET GOING WITH YOUR DREAMS

There is a significant relationship between how you move your body and the way you feel emotionally. Furthermore, there is a significant relationship between how you feel emotionally and the level of success that you achieve.

One of the philosophies that I live and base my life on is....

... that success comes from liking the way you feel about something - and how you feel is a result of the way you move your body.

The word 'emotion' comes from the Latin word 'movere', which means 'to move'. This is no coincidence. Therefore, the way you feel, your emotion, comes from the way you use your body. Emotion is, in fact, motion.

So the truth is that even though we are all from different places in the world, and are different shapes and sizes, have different levels of health and financial wealth and practise different religions - and providing we are not physically or mentally impaired in some serious way - we all have and share the same emotional capacity.

In short, we all have the same ability to feel happiness, sadness, joy, pain, laughter, love, loneliness, pride, shame, courage and passion and so on.

This is my first key message to you in this book - if you use your body in certain ways then you will feel better and will achieve more.

The way you use your body - your breathing, posture, stance, the way you talk, the way you walk and the tension in your muscles - all make a difference to the way you feel.

Think of the way you use your body when you're happy, excited, proud, celebrating, sad or angry. You breathe in a different way and have different amounts of tension in your muscles when you are angry compared to when you feel a sense of pride. If you are angry and you make a conscious effort to change the way and depth of your breathing, your feelings of anger will lessen.

This means that we choose and create the way that we feel. We are not victims of circumstance: what we do physically affects the way we feel so we can actually condition ourselves to feel more of what we want to feel.

However, being in poor health puts you at a severe disadvantage with regard to this. If you don't take care of your body – by being overweight, for example - it's tough to have a lot of energy on a consistent basis. To be able to express full joy, full happiness and full vitality you need to have good health and vibrancy. If you don't, you're only going to be able to express 50%, for example, rather than 100% of who you really are.

So if how you use your body is so important to what you achieve and how you feel, it follows then that you should take good care of your body. It is the 'vessel' through which you're going to express, experience and feel everything. You're going to feel every emotion through it. Everything you're going to express and every message you're going to put across is going to come from this vessel.

Your body is what you use to get you through life. If you use it properly you can achieve all the things that you want to achieve in life. When your body is being taken care of, your true abilities and your spirit can shine through. On the other hand, not taking care of this gift of life will get in the way of your success.

So this is my second message - look after your body.

There are ways of taking care of your body that really work and I will go through those with you in this book.

My third key message is that actions speak louder than words.

In the past I have sat and spoken to people and of course, had some impact on their lives, but the biggest reactions I have ever received have been from the things that I have actually *physically done*. When people have come up to me and said that they have been inspired by me it's always been because of the energy I have put out or actions I have taken.

Over the years I have read many personal development books. I learned a great deal from them; however, having read them I'd fall short of real success because what I learned only made sense in my head. It was only on the occasions that I 'owned' the messages by getting them into my body that I'd get the successes promised by the authors 100%.

This paralleled my show business career. Everything I've ever achieved was because I owned it in my body. I expressed it always in auditions, castings and on stage. Often without saying a word the emotional transference came through loud and clear.

In the past, I hadn't been the best of speakers, due to my lack of a wide vocabulary. But somehow I always had lots of friends and many people admired and respected me. Also I was often asked to hold responsible positions such as school prefect and team captain. So something about me was coming across to people, although not in words.

What I've come to realise is that it was the way I held myself and the emotions that I put across that made the impact on people. Actions have always been my biggest selling point.

Although I'm now conscious of the fact, I've realised that so many people are just not aware of their biggest communication tool – their physical body. I've observed business people, for example, searching so hard for the right words to make the right impression when all they had to do was adopt the right physiology.

Of course this is no surprise as we have all been conditioned to communicate verbally. When I think back to my school days, the way things would work is that we'd all sit there passively and listen to the teacher just talk and talk and talk. They'd drone on and on and not hold my attention at all. However, whenever we had a teacher that made things more interactive I remembered much more. When I used my body and not just my ears in the learning process I absorbed so much more information.

It wasn't until recently that I discovered that scientists have done work that supports this. A study conducted in 1967 by psychologist Albert Mehrabian set out to distinguish the importance of verbal and nonverbal communication. The conclusion he reached was that 7% of communication is verbal, 38% is vocal (that is, tone of voice, volume, pace, etc) and 55% is via your face and physiology.

The latest and most effective learning method is known as accelerated learning. What it involves is not listening passively to what is being said as, in that instance, you only retain about 8-12% of what you hear. If you take some notes the retention rate increases to 50%. But if you make notes, engage all your senses and get actively involved in a physical way then your muscles and nervous system experience the learning material as a form of muscle memory. When this happens your level of retention rises to almost 95%.

Learning dance combinations illustrates this point so well. When practising and performing you put so much into your body and feel the emotion that goes with the routine at a deep level. In the end it is conditioned into your nervous system so that years later you can do the routine again like second nature.

As a dancer, I discovered my ability to feel and express myself emotionally in ways that I hadn't done previously. It was as if I had been cut off from certain emotions or didn't feel I could express them even though they were there. But through movement and the exploration of dance, I gained the ability to access powerful emotions, such as passion, drive, courage, grace, determination, compassion, humility, elegance and love.

As a dancer I often feel like an artist painting a fluid sculpture: whatever moves I make allow me to experience yet another emotion. Think of all the great people who have moved us in magnificent ways through such endeavours as sports, music, dance and the arts. They all find unique ways to use their physiology to touch, move and inspire us to use our own physiology.

This book will expose you to the amazing possibilities of the human physiology. With what I teach you, you'll be able to consistently emanate the right energy and emotion and take in and absorb information to the maximum. You'll be able to express yourself fully by linking everything to the way you feel.

My final key message is the crucial importance of moving for success.

What I have discovered over many years is that most people do know what to do to improve and get the results they want. They do know that they should, for example, take more care of their health, really communicate with their partner and be more courageous. They *know* all these things. They *know* but they don't *do*.

What I've experienced through dance is that it's always stretched me. Knowing how to do a move doesn't help. You can watch someone else do it and ask your teacher questions until you're blue in the face but the bottom line is that the only way you can do it is to get out there onto the floor and do it. If you want to execute five pirouettes you've got to get up and physically do pirouettes. One, one-two, one-two-three, one-two-three-four, one-two-three-four and then five. You actually physically do it until you get to the point where you do five and can honestly say, "I can really do this".

I've achieved many dreams in the world of dance. For years I appeared in my dream part in the musical that I always wanted to be in - Electra in Starlight Express. Dreaming was one thing but I had to take action. The only way to get to my goal was to keep taking action until I got there.

WHAT I LEARNED FROM MADONNA

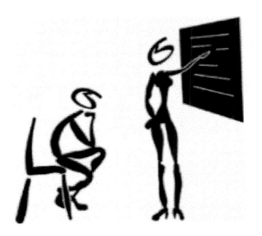

As I said at the start of this book, I have been very privileged because I have had some great teachers. I want to make a special mention of one of them because she epitomizes what this book is about – getting into action and going after your dreams. That's what Madonna has done all her life.

She said once that she's not the greatest singer or dancer but she is a very convincing artist. I observed how she used her body in such beautiful and unique ways. It was something that transferred to all who were near or around her.

I was always amazed and intrigued from just watching her in videos or on TV. Of course such performances can always be enhanced and manipulated through the use of lights and special effects. But it was when I witnessed her 'live and direct' so to speak that I became fully convinced of her expertise and talents.

It was a remarkable experience to be in the same room as her. Her movements and actions allow you to experience what was truly going on in her world. Her feelings, dreams and expectations are right there in the way in which she moves.

She has the ability to lift you to a point where you expect more of yourself. She has a background in dance and is completely in touch with her body and its capabilities and this is something that she explores to the max.

She expresses so much emotion in the way that she moves. She generates so much energy, be it sensual, powerful, graceful or dynamic. It is so magical and phenomenal to be around.

You can see her ability to continually reinvent herself due to the flexibility of her movement. This enhances the range of emotion she allows herself to experience and allows her to be able to adapt to so many different styles. This versatility is one of the key secrets to life as it allows you to keep diversifying, exploring, learning and experiencing something new. It allows you to keep growing.

I spent a whole weekend working with her to rehearse and perform a dance routine. It's very apparent why she is such a star. The energy she puts into her work is phenomenal. The first time I met her she said this is what I do.

She didn't do a half-hearted walk-through as most people would have done in that situation. She did a full-on show. The way she spoke and explained things was so profound and she spoke with such spirit, panache and self-assurance. I was in complete admiration of her courage, boldness and daring.

She would put so much into the rehearsals and would have swum 40 lengths before she'd even arrived at the dance studios in the morning. The rehearsal process was so profound. She has an exceptionally high standard and is so driven. She'd make sure we kept working until the routine was exactly how she wanted it to be.

She was that way about everything. We rehearsed and rehearsed and rehearsed and she would give 100% each and every time. I was so influenced by her energy because she was giving so much and the rehearsal routines were so powerful. So when it came to the show itself it was just amazing.

Being with her for that whole weekend was a phenomenal experience. Nothing was too much trouble. Her entourage was on hand the whole time to make sure that everything ran smoothly.

She has a real presence about her. It's the way she walks and carries herself generally. She is someone that knows what she wants and will do what is necessary to make it a reality. Because of the amount of energy she puts out, that comes back tenfold.

When I worked with her she was 10 years into her career and she'd made it. She was then, and probably still is a number one female music star. She still takes care of her body and that movement is still a big part of who she is as a performer. She is always a delight to watch. She could have taken it easy but she wanted to give her best in every way, shape or form. It was extraordinary to witness first hand. Her identity is that way. She is a star to the core of her being.

She just raised the level of performance of everyone that was involved. For example, lighting and sound guys are used to cues to turn lights on or off, for example, that are really easy to pick up. But Madonna wanted things to be very, very precise. For example, she'd say that she wanted a light to turn on when she sang a particular word. I thought there was no way the guys would be able to work in that way but they did.

She wouldn't accept poor performance and because of how and who she was people stepped up their game. She makes things happen around her.

When she says we need to do whatever it takes to get the results she wants, she really means it.

So if until this point in your life you've talked a good talk but not really got anywhere, then this book is for you. I will show you how you can truly walk your talk and do what you've got to do.

The lesson I learned from that experience is that when you move well you move people.

MY JOURNEY BEGINS: FROM ELECTRICIAN TO ELECTRA

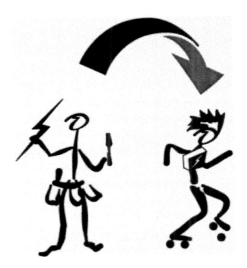

I wasn't consciously aware of the principles I will teach in this book when I was realising my dream of appearing in Starlight Express. It was only when I looked back at what I did and examined what other people who have achieved their dreams had done – for example, Madonna – that I noticed the patterns.

Stories are a wonderful way of teaching messages. My intention in relating how I achieved one of my dreams is not to impress you, but to illustrate that if I - a one-time shy apprentice electrician - can go from nowhere to appearing for over 10 years in one of the top musicals of all time, then so can you achieve whatever your dream is. As you read my story look for the lessons and I will expand on them in later chapters.

My dream of appearing as Electra in Starlight Express started in 1986 when a friend, George, actually got into the West

End show. He often said that if I ever wanted to come, just to let him know. I always said that I'd come and see him one day but would put it to the back of my mind each time.

A little while later, I was pursuing a really nice girl and decided to take George up on his offer. I kept seeing her in class and decided to ask her if she liked going to the theatre. Starlight was a really hit show by this point so when I said that I could get a pair of tickets she was really impressed!

George had told me that he was in the show but he hadn't really explained what the show was like or what he was doing within it. Up until this point I'd never been to a theatre before.

So when it came to the big night I was like a little child walking into the auditorium. I was expecting something traditional. For example, when the curtains were raised I expected to see the cast simply skating around on stage. But I was amazed at how the entire auditorium was the set.

I was in such awe before the show had started and then the first number just completely blew me away. I totally forgot that I was even on a date!

I was just so mesmerised by the trains coming out of the tunnel. Suddenly you just saw these train lights coming from nowhere. I thought it was amazing. That aspect of the show just really held me - the power of those trains!

Then halfway through the show something happened. **The next character to appear on stage was about to change my life.** There was what seemed like an electrical fault, and then suddenly from nowhere this bridge somehow appeared. It reminded me of something out of Star Trek. It planted itself on the stage and this guy, who looked as if he came out of the back of the wall, just appeared there. It was Electra. The Electric Train. The train of the future.

There was something special for me about that character, Electra. The person playing the part was truly phenomenal. He was strong, confident, tall, sexy, robotic, unpredictable, charismatic, a leader emanating pure, passionate energy. It was Tom Jobe who played that part and he was just amazing - his character and everything about the way he moved. I totally related to the way he did things.

I knew in the core of my being that I must perform this part in this show.

Electra was very versatile and adaptable. He kept changing and I could completely relate to that. At the time, I loved the fact that I was doing different styles of dance in my classes. The Electra character's versatility reminded me of my boyhood hero, the magically gifted and versatile footballer George Best, a man who could play anywhere on the football pitch, with such grace and flexibility and skill.

Electra would switch from being very robotic to being very fluid. From being feminine to masculine. He was all these things in one character. I was simply hypnotised and said to myself: 'I've got to play that part. That's a role I must play.'

But how can I play it? It was of course the high and mighty, professional West End. I had no Actor's Equity Card, something at that time that was very hard to attain. I hadn't had a singing lesson in my life. How was this going to happen? Just knowing that this role was so much a part of who I am, I automatically took the necessary steps.

I was twenty one years of age and thoughts like "I don't know how, but I have to play that role" and "Electra is just me" kept on running through my head as I sat there and watched the show for the first time.

Electra was like a magnet. I was hypnotised every time he came on stage. My eyes were drawn to this character. Tom Jobe was simply amazing.

The show I saw had pretty much the opening night cast, although Tom had taken over as Electra from Jeffrey Daniels who left after six months.

My friend George was the Japanese train. He was an amazing skater and he was perfect for that role as he could tumble and do all sorts of tricks. He was just dynamite but it was Electra that was my perfect part.

From that first moment on, the show really mesmerized me. I asked George if could come again and again and I was going as often as I possibly could.

I lost count of how many times I went and seeing my friend George really gave me a buzz. And seeing George being in the show got me thinking I could realise my dream too. After all, he didn't have an Equity Card. He was a dancer/skater but somehow he got in the show and learned singing while there.

So, I went and practised roller skating in my local park as often as possible. I asked George to get me the words from Electra's main song, so I could practise with the CD of the show. I went to singing lessons. I owned this part. Often at home I would perform the part in the mirror.

George is one of those guys that really loves skating and wherever he goes he takes his roller skates with him. He was in the studio one day and was just skating around and, as luck would have it, one of the assistant choreographers from Starlight just happened to be in the studio. She was really impressed and asked him if he'd like to go for an audition.

George wasn't sure. The show was just starting out and they needed really strong skaters. When he told me he was going for an audition I remember I was so sceptical. He was taken on to be a support but went straight into the show.

After I'd been to see the show a few times I decided that if I was going to succeed I'd need to become a strong skater as well as an exceptional dancer. So I started skating literally every day. I started to take my skates everywhere just like George.

It wasn't long, as far as I was concerned, before I could have played that role there and then. I was ready in my mind. If I could have talked to the choreographer I'd have said: "Just give me the costume, I can do it now."

But I had no clue about singing the right notes and harmonies at that point. I could play the part and that is all I could see in my mind. I related to and identified with Electra 100% and that was all there was to it.

At that point I was telling everybody I wanted to be in the show but did not reveal which role. It was only if someone said to me that I'd make a good Electra that I'd admit that that was the part I wanted to play.

I got positive feedback. Many people said that the show was totally me and that they could envisage me in it. No-one told me I was crazy because the people I was mixing with at the time were all young, keen and eager to get on in show business themselves.

I was doing the whole Flashdance thing at the time. I was an electrician by day and dancing at night. I was leaving the house at six in the morning and getting home at ten at night. I was going straight from work to the dance classes. And I was doing that five days a week and still going to dance classes at the weekend.

When I started at the beginner classes I felt good being around these people. Then I realised that if I wanted to be better I'd have to get out of the comfort zone and go to a higher class. I knew being with an intermediate level group of people would push me higher and I remember seeing advanced professional classes and thinking, one day soon, I'll be there.

For me it took guts to progress to intermediate classes. These people weren't professional but they were good and I had to produce to match them. I didn't want to look stupid after all! I was beginning to realize that being around the right people takes you higher.

At that point I didn't have an interest in musicals and dance generally. Anything to do with show business was worlds away. I thought that was for rich people only. It was not something I felt I had any connection with.

I grew up in Ealing, London and was just your regular kid. I did all the things that boys do. I played football, went fishing, rode bicycles and all the other normal things that ordinary kids do.

My father was a meat inspector and my mother was a domestic assistant at a hospital. My brother was a car mechanic and my sister a nurse. In our world it was all about just getting yourself a good job.

And that's what I did. I became an apprentice electrician and did all those regular things that you do when you get your first job. I mixed with the lads, went to the pub, played pool and became part of that whole scene.

I remember before I started as an electrician the careers advice woman had asked me what I'd like to do and I didn't know. I told her that I liked figuring out how things work and she suggested becoming an electrician. And that was it. I became an electrician.

So here I was a few years on from that chat with the careers officer - an electrician by day and a dance student at night. Unhappy with my day job, I was waiting for my big break in dance to come along before I signed off my career as an electrician.

And then a point came where I just decided that I was going to leave. The guys I was working with were all in their forties and fifties. They'd tell me stories about what they did when they were young. They were doing my job now and I thought to myself: "I've got no stories to tell and if I don't do something with my life I won't have any stories to tell my children when I'm older."

I began to think that being an electrician wasn't my world any more. Their conversations were boring and depressing to me now. In dance I was discovering more opportunities to express myself. In this world I was meeting people who were more animated and open and always happy to see me. It was in sharp contrast to what I was used to but I was relating more and more to this world.

So one day I just handed my notice in and was gone within a week. I knew I could always come back and be an electrician again. I would have just lived a bit of life in the meantime.

I was now a full-time, professional dancer! The first job I actually got was pantomime in Reading and I got to work with Mr Sulu from Star Trek. I was working with a choreographer I had worked with before and she made me her assistant to the choreography. A great start. It was a fantastic experience and the great thing about it was that it was a three month job, from rehearsals in November through to January.

The really spooky thing is how often Starlight Express would pop into my world even at that early point in my new career. Strange coincidences were happening. I would be rehearsing for something else and they would be rehearsing for Starlight next door, for example.

There was one occasion when I was working for the Lenny Henry TV show. In one sketch we were doing a take-off of Michael Jackson's *Bad* video.

One scene needed someone to roller skate and I volunteered. Rehearsing next door were the cast from Starlight and I kept hoping that someone would wander in from there, notice me doing my routine and ask me to do an audition on the spot.

I did audition for Starlight in 1986 long before I actually made it. On that first occasion I was doing some TV work at the time with Dougie Squires, the choreographer. We were rehearsing and the Starlight audition was right in the middle of one of the rehearsal sessions. I asked Dougie if I could take some time off to go and he said it wouldn't be fair to everybody else if I were to go. The TV show we were doing was going to be recorded the following day. I knew all my steps and, in the end, we didn't actually do any dancing in the afternoon but sat down and just did a read through of the songs.

Fortunately, though, the Starlight people said they were willing to give me a private audition because I couldn't make the main one. I thought that was great because I wouldn't be one of many but would have the whole stage to myself.

So off I went to the audition. I had the worst audition I had done in my whole career. I did really appallingly. The problem was that although I could roller skate and I could dance, I couldn't do both together! I couldn't execute any of the steps they asked of me - and that wasn't many! Executing moves on skates was a whole new concept.

So the creative team just said thank you very much, and I left. I went home completely disheartened. It was just the worst I could have done, in my opinion. But within a few hours of getting home they called and said they'd like to see me again. They must have seen something there. They said that they would like to see me at the recalls at a later date. I couldn't believe it. Maybe they did notice the performer in me through that disaster of an audition. I jumped and celebrated like crazy. I was back on track. All I needed to do was master the steps I had destroyed in the first audition and I'd be fine. Or so I thought. The next audition was even harder than the first.

There were a lot of people at the recall session but I thought I'd be OK because I felt ready. But what happened was a shock to us all. We started out by doing that routine but then they got us to play the toughest part physically from the show - the character of Rocky.

It involves doing a lot of acrobatics and tricks. All of a sudden this was the level of the audition. I fell about fifteen times. It was just a mess. Apart from a couple of guys everyone was doing as badly, though.

I finished off by singing an Elvis number and although I'd never sung in public before I saw a smile in the choreographer's eyes and I left the room with some hope.

I wasn't really familiar with singing exact notes, keys and harmonies but I thought I'd done OK. However, when I heard the guy that followed me in sing, I knew that he was in a different league from me at the time. Within a few days I heard that he was in the show.

They told me I'd done well and to try again because they refresh the cast once a year. Occasionally they would have in-between auditions if somebody didn't make it or if they needed extra people.

So I had a year to practise. And practise I did. I really worked at it. I went back again for auditions but still didn't make it.

Then in 1987 a new opportunity came up to join the show that would tour Japan and Australia, two places I'd love to visit doing my dream show. What an opportunity that was. They had a succession of auditions for the show over a three month period.

By that point I was so 'on it' as far as auditioning for the show was concerned. I had auditioned it so much that the choreography was in my bones.

For the final audition I had one of those days when everything was just there. I was in the zone and every spin I did and every move I executed was exactly right on the count. I didn't fall and didn't slip and all the other fellow auditioners applauded when I finished.

But I still didn't get in. I just couldn't believe it. I searched for what could be missing with what I was doing. All they said to me was that I should keep practising my skating and to try again the following year. But I saw other people get in who couldn't skate as well as me so I began to get a bit despondent at this point. I began to think it wasn't meant to be and the whole idea of getting into Starlight started to wane.

It was at this point where I was thinking it just wasn't going to happen for me that I came across an ad in *The Stage* newspaper for a huge audition for Starlight Express in Germany. It didn't really excite me though. I just thought to myself that they'd seen me audition so many times that if they wanted me they'd have hired me by now.

And then something really spooky happened. A tiny twist of fate was about to change my life again. I went to my regular dance class in Covent Garden one day. I always wear an elastic belt to keep up my trousers in class. However, on this particular day I'd forgotten it. I had a few minutes before my class started so I decided to run into the shop next door to buy another one. And who should I bump into in there but Arlene Phillips, the famous choreographer who had turned me down all those times for Starlight in London.

She asked how I was doing and what I was up to. I said I was doing fine and that I was doing bits and bobs here and there. Then she dropped a bombshell. "How would you like to go to Germany to do Starlight Express?", she said. "Do you mean an audition?" I replied. "No, I want you to do it," she answered.

Wow! Straight into the show. I just couldn't believe it. She told me to think about it overnight and to call her the next day. This was the Tuesday and they were flying out to Germany on the Sunday.

It seemed they just needed more people. I was going to be an understudy. I didn't realize it at the time but they needed strong covers for the three Rocky parts in particular, which are physically very demanding. People playing one of the Rocky parts are often injured.

I told all my friends and they told me that this was a huge opportunity. They told me that I just had to do it. In fact, they were more excited than I was for some reason that I couldn't explain.

I spoke to my family and they told me that this was a big Andrew Lloyd Webber show and that I should go for it. My girlfriend supported me and also said I should go as it was only an hour away and I could fly back often.

However, I wasn't sure about flying out to start a year-long stint on the show at such short notice. So in the morning I rang Arlene and asked if I could come out in a couple of weeks. Arlene was great as she said that I could fly out in a fortnight and could catch up with rehearsals. This all happened in March and they were due to open on May 28 so there was time for me to get up to speed.

So finally I picked up my one-way ticket and I was off. Until that point London had been my life as I had never lived anywhere else.

I was 25 years of age and couldn't speak a word of German. And suddenly here I was with a one-way ticket and a pair of roller skates over my shoulder on my way to a whole new world.

Somebody met me at the airport and took me to my hotel room in Hamburg. It was a tiny room. I was told to sign my name on all these forms and I had no clue exactly what I was signing.

I was told to make my way to the bus station in the morning and to look out for the other guys from the team. She said that it would be obvious who they were because they would be the only ones who would have roller skates hanging over their shoulders. We'd all then be able to travel to the rehearsals together.

After she'd gone I just remember sitting in this hotel room thinking "What am I doing here?" It all seemed so crazy. I didn't know anyone and I didn't speak the language. That first morning I took a walk around the city. It was so strange to me. The only thing I knew how to do was to buy a kebab!

It was late winter and the weather was cold and dreary. Hamburg was like a cleaner version of London though. My hotel room was clean and everything was so well organised.

I didn't enjoy my first morning of rehearsals. I sat alone and didn't know anyone. In fact the choreographer didn't even introduce me to the rest of the company. All she said to me was 'That's the person you have got to follow and watch what he does'.

Fortunately, however, I was soon able to make some friends. Dawn, my girlfriend at the time, knew some members of the cast so I didn't feel completely alone for long.

It was a really multinational class. There were Germans, Americans, Danish, Australians, New Zealanders, Austrian, Dutch, Swiss and British people. There were 40 of us in total: 25 on stage and the rest understudies and back ups. Starlight Express is very demanding physically so a large number of back ups are required.

The first thing I looked for was to see who was playing Electra. I saw that he was tall like myself so I felt good about that. He was pretty good. In fact, he was more than that - he was an amazing Electra. My contract mentioned playing the parts of the engines, the Rockies and the components. The part of Electra was not mentioned and the choreographer, Arlene Phillips, had no clue that I wanted to play Electra.

The rehearsals for the show were very intense and demanding. There were days when my entire body was completely numb. It was as if we were simultaneously training to run the marathon and the 100 metres sprint at the Olympics whilst singing at the top of our voices. The show was of an amazingly high standard. We were pushed and stretched to the maximum. The intense training was necessary because we were expected to perform eight shows a week.

I don't know why but in life I've always seemed to have had the ability to move up the ranks quite quickly into some sort of leadership role. The same happened with Starlight. For example, I became the first understudy to appear on stage. I'd arrived at the rehearsals last of all and suddenly I was the first out of fifteen understudies to get to be on stage. Firstly, I became one of the four Rockies and within months I was playing Rocky One.

Opening night was put back a couple of weeks because the sets weren't workable. They had to build different banks and the show finally opened on June 12th.

The show had a week of previews and there were standing ovations for each one. We all knew it was going to be a big success. It was a success in London and this show was twice as spectacular. The stage was huge, the costumes were amazing plus the lighting and lasers were outstanding.

The theatre was simply ideal for Starlight Express. Bochum is a provincial town and people were saying that they didn't believe it would work because it was a small town compared to other German cities. But they were proved wrong. Coaches were coming in every day from all over Germany, Austria and Switzerland. Up until that point all the shows such as Cats and Phantom Of The Opera had played in Hamburg.

Very soon I was doing a lot of understudying. And what began to happen is that the more times I understudied the more often they would use me to understudy. They were playing safe and did not want to risk bringing in a new substitute when they knew that I was up to the job.

I soon realized that there were only two Electra covers in the house and they were both actually first cast people. So, in fact, none of the covers for Electra were backstage people. So I suggested to the management people that they could use me as cover for Electra. They responded by saying that my singing wasn't very strong and that the part demanded good singing ability.

So I suggested that they make me emergency cover and give me some singing lessons. I told them that I wasn't expecting them to pay me for understudying Electra but, if they could support me in my singing lessons, that I just wanted to be emergency cover for Electra. They agreed so I was yet another step closer to playing Electra.

So I started in rehearsals as Electra. It was all very strange because I was learning the part in German. I started to get into the feel of the part. I was relating to Electra. I learnt the lines in no time at all because I was watching it every night. Learning the choreography also was easy, because I was so eager and enthusiastic. It was going straight into my body. Every so often we'd do run-throughs of the show and I'd get very positive comments.

People would say to me: "Wow, I didn't know you could do that". The truth was that people were really in awe of the way I did it. My voice still wasn't 100% and that had to be improved.

I hadn't mastered all the notes and harmonies. I have a bass baritone voice; some of Electra's singing was written quite high.

They were making allowances for me as far my singing was concerned. Of course this wasn't ideal because I wasn't singing in the way that Andrew Lloyd Webber had intended his songs to be sung.

This was quite frustrating for me. I really wanted to sing that part the way it was meant to be sung. So I kept on practising. The last run-through I had was in January 1989. They told me that they were getting by really well with the covers they had and had no need for me right now as emergency cover.

I was so disappointed but my big break came in May 1989. There was a cast changeover and those covers were leaving and new people were coming in.

Very soon there was unrest amongst the new cast. The management were unhappy with the actor playing "CB", one of the lead roles. They weren't putting him on and were going with his understudy instead. The lead was very unhappy and he was in real conflict with the management team. The actor playing Electra got wind of this. He did not have a cover and threatened that he would not go on in support of his friend.

This was all getting out of control because suddenly they had nobody to play Electra, one of the lead roles. As for the actor playing CB, he could sing and dance but they weren't happy with him.

The start time of the show was 8pm, and at five minutes to eight one night Electra announced that he was not going to go on stage in protest at the way his friend was being treated. I was in my Rocky make-up with five minutes to go until the curtains opened.

I was called into the office to be told that they wanted me to play Electra. I was torn inside: I was excited but scared at the same time. They asked if I could do it and in a split second I replied that I could. I had no time to think.

Fortunately Electra doesn't go on until twenty minutes into the show. I had to quickly change my make-up and costume. I had directions being fired at me as lines and harmonies buzzed around in my head.

I had to do it. I just had to. There was no way I could say no to this big chance and let them down. So twenty five minutes later there I was standing on the bridge on the set from where Electra makes his entrance.

Electra stands on the bridge with his back to the audience. There is a build up to this entrance and then suddenly Electra slides down the slope in a dramatic way announcing, "I am Electric".

Before I went for it I had to really get myself into the right emotional state and do some deep breathing and then, 'whoosh', I just went for it. There I was performing my dream part in front an appreciative audience of two thousand people. It was just an unbelievable experience.

When I finished that first number I had a feeling of ecstasy. I'd finally made it. I'd finally done it. I hadn't had a rehearsal since January and here I was in June but I was just completely confident. I was in the zone just doing everything perfectly. I said to myself: "This is my part. It's always been my part."

Although I hadn't had a formal rehearsal for months, believe me, I had been practising. I'd been practising in my mind for years and I'd physically been rehearsing in my hotel room every day I'd been in Germany. I played the soundtrack CD all the time. I was practising my singing for Electra, practising and just plain living as Electra. I was Electra!

THE POWER TO MOVE FOR SUCCESS

HOW TO STOP WHAT'S BEEN STOPPING YOU FROM MOVING FORWARD

IT'S ALL ABOUT FEAR

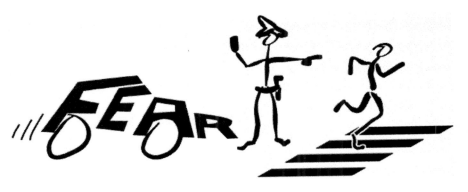

I had a coaching client once who was in a very unhappy relationship. In fact, the relationship bordered on being abusive.

She felt like her needs were not being met. If she had left that relationship she would, of course, have become available for the right kind of partner. But she stayed in the bad relationship nonetheless even though doing so was a tremendous strain on her energies.

Sometimes she'd say to me that she'd tell her partner it was all over that upcoming weekend. On the Monday I'd check in and she'd give me excuses. She'd say, "He was nicer this weekend" or "It just wasn't the right time because he was in a bad mood" or would come up with some other similar excuse.

"Fear does not have any special power unless you empower it by submitting to it."
- Les Brown, Author and Speaker

From talking to her I found that, at a deeper level, what was really holding her back was fear. She was scared to end the relationship. She was scared of being alone. "Who else would entertain having me if I finish this relationship now?", she'd say.

In my show business career I've always wanted things so much that I overcame the fear. Auditioning for a part you really want in front of a panel who are just there to judge you, is scary. You're putting yourself on the line but because that's an unavoidable part of the process, you blast through the fear. If I want something badly enough I don't care how silly, crazy or mad I have to be to get what I want, I'll do it.

People don't take the action they need to take to get what they want because of fear. But if you take the action the fear goes.

People imagine the nasty consequences that might result from taking action. In all my experience I have never met anyone who conquered fears and said that what happened was bad.

The truth is that everything you really want in life is on the other side of fear. You can't get away from fear. It will always be there, but it's how you handle it that matters.

At the root of all our fears is our basic instinct to protect ourselves. We are programmed to respond when faced with danger.

The basic reaction to threats is known as the 'fight or flight' response. When it is set off the body responds in a very particular way:

-   the face muscles tense up

- muscles freeze
- the heart rate speeds up
- blood pressure rises
- breathing becomes shallow and slow

The purpose of this 'freezing up' of the body is to provide time for the mind to decide on the best course of action. It prepares the body to either fight the danger head on or to run away depending on what the brain decides is the best way forward.

This survival instinct serves us well except when it kicks in at the wrong time and stops us from moving towards what we really want. The problem is that in our modern world, fear rears its head in the face of both real and imagined dangers.

With your fears and phobias you'll find that you are not afraid of the thing itself, but are actually afraid of either:

- losing or not having control; or
- not being good enough to cope

The situation will only be what you perceive the situation to be. Therefore, what you fear is your own perception of reality. For example, if you have a phobia about open spaces, logically you know that there is little to fear. It is your perception of the situation that is the problem. You do not want to go out because you do not want to feel the sense of fear that you think you will have. Your perception is that you will lose control and you are fearful of that.

This way of thinking probably permeates through to all that you want to do in life but are afraid to do and that is a problem that you must overcome.

OVERCOME FEAR WITH COURAGE

"Courage is mastery of fear, not absence of fear."
- Mark Twain

The definition of courage is feeling fear but then doing what has to be done nonetheless. There's an old saying that cowards feel fear 40 times, whereas courageous people feel fear only once.

Courage is the ability to act in spite of the fear. To get your goals you have to take the steps necessary.

When I was a young boy I didn't learn to swim. It wasn't a problem until one year when I was going to go on holiday to Italy with a bunch of lads. I knew we'd hang around the pool a lot and realised it would be really embarrassing if I couldn't swim. I just knew I had to learn to swim before we went.

This was a big fear for me but I knew I had to conquer it if I wanted to enjoy the holiday. What I decided to do was to tackle the challenge head-on.

One day I took myself off to the local leisure centre and went to a section of the swimming pool where I knew I could stand up. I was as scared as hell but jumped in nonetheless. I took a deep breath in and pushed myself off from the side of the pool. I just kicked and splashed away and then something happened. I just found motion.

I had faith that if I kicked my legs and moved my arms that something good would happen. I swam for the first time in my life. That was a really courageous thing for me to do because I didn't have a teacher. I just went for it. I knew what I wanted and I was prepared to do what was necessary to make it happen.

The word courage comes from the French word, coeur, which means heart. So when you are being courageous what you're doing is coming from the heart. An act of courage is the heart overriding the head. Fears are in your head and courage is in your heart.

What you really want to do is stored in your heart. The courageous thing seems illogical to the rational mind. The mind says, "Why do something that is dangerous?"

But the truth is that to get to where you want to in life you need to do the courageous thing.

That does not mean you should be foolhardy and reckless. It means that you should listen to your heart and, if a goal feels right to you, then you should follow your heart. Do whatever is necessary, no matter how seemingly ridiculous, to get to what you want.

Fear is a real immobiliser although it does have its place. We're born with just a few basic fears and the rest we just make up. It's right to be fearful of a tiger, for example. The 'fight or flight' response is in-built into our nervous systems, but most of our fears are ego-driven.

I'd put the fear of rejection and the fear of failure into this category. They really hold people back. They're ego-driven because they're about not wanting to look bad or feel embarrassed. At the root of these ego-driven fears are the feelings of not being good enough and being out of control.

Everyone feels fear no matter who they are or what they've achieved in life. And, in fact, some people - not wanting to be considered a coward - give their fears different names such as apprehension or stress. But call these feelings what you like, they're still fears.

JUST DO IT

Stress means that you don't have a grip on the situation you find yourself in. Whole books have been written and day-long seminars have been run trying to teach people how to conquer fears, but how to do it can be summed up in five simple words – just do what you fear. That, my friends, is it.

If you're scared of heights climb to the top of your nearest mountain. If you're scared of lifts then get in one. You can do hours of therapy but you won't actually conquer your fear until you do it. Nothing happens until that.

Reality is only our perception. If you fear open spaces and I don't, it doesn't mean that you are right to be scared or that I am right not to be. It's about perception but if you change that perception then that fear disappears for you.

If you feared flying you could conquer that fear by 'modelling' the pilot who flies on planes everyday. Modelling meaning that you'd adopt a pilot's entire physiology and thoughts – do that, and you'd get the job done.

However, if you walked onto the plane apprehensively then you'd be frightened out of your life. Let your body lead the way and your mind will follow.

Stars manage their physiology successfully during performances. Thousands of kids all over the country can sing a ten-out-of-ten performance in the safety of their bedrooms but put them in front of a large audience and most flunk it. Stars don't, though – it's when the stage is the biggest that they perform at their best. They put themselves into the right stance, create the right tension in their body, breathe in the necessary way, go into a 'zone' and feed off the crowds. Often performers will tell you that they were nervous during a performance, but they used their bodies in ways that changed that nervous feeling to deliver confidence during the performance.

Why should anyone fear public speaking, for example? Think about it. Physically all that's involved is standing up and talking - something which people do many times a day. What's different with public speaking, of course, is that there is an audience - and it's the judgements of that audience that people fear.

Fear is the enemy of success. It can paralyze you from taking action. At the root of fear is our basic instinct for survival. When the brain senses fear, it sends messages to the body to move into fight-or-flight mode. This triggers physiological changes – the heart rate speeds up, blood pressure rises and breathing becomes shallow and fast. Although the body is, at this moment, surging with adrenaline it freezes to allow time for the brain to decide on the best course of action. The choices are to stay and fight the apparent danger or to flee the scene.

These instinctive responses exist to protect us from the many dangerous life-threatening situations that are all around us. Otherwise, we would all walk across the path of speeding cars on the motorway. So although essential for survival, fear can become a problem if it stops us moving towards what we really want.

There is an acronym for the word fear which I don't subscribe to - Forget Everything And Run! One that I do think is spot on, though, is False Evidence that Appears Real.

If you encounter a hungry tiger then you have every right to believe that your fear is justified. However, if your fear is of asking someone you really like out on a date, then it is out of place. People ask people out for dates all the time and it is not a life-threatening thing to do. The fear is based on perceptions of the situation.

Fears that paralyze us to take action towards what we want in life are called ego-based fears. They include fear of failure, rejection, embarrassment, looking stupid and even fear of success.

THE CONQUERING FEARS EXERCISE:

1. *The key to conquering fears is to put yourself into a courageous state as often as possible. You do this through the way you use your body, controlling your focus and using positive inner talk. Successful people are that way because they do this. You should seek to condition this courageous state into your being.*

2. *Always remember that courage is the ability to act in spite of the fear. On the other side of the fear is freedom. Courage is the most important virtue because without it you achieve nothing.*

3. *Rehearse situations in your mind that you fear such as asking someone out and being turned down - but change the response you'd normally give in that situation to a positive one. So say, for example, you get an answer back such as: "No I don't want to go out with you because I'm not attracted to you". You should practise giving a confident reply such as: "Oh, that's a shame because we would have been so good together. Your loss."*

4. *Focus solely on the outcomes and rewards that you want from fearful situations. Link in your mind as much pleasure as you can to the reward and as much discomfort or pain as you can to not crossing through the fear. Feel a real sense of passion and desire for what you really want.*

THE STEPS THAT WILL GET YOU MOVING

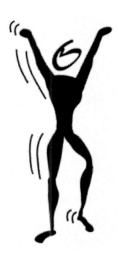

There are people who tell me that they really want a luxury house overlooking the sea or a speedboat or a Porsche. I ask them if they really want those things because they don't seem to take any action towards getting the things they say they want.

So do you really want what you think you want?

TRULY IDENTIFY WITH YOUR GOALS

"I am the greatest. I predicted being the heavyweight champion of the world by the end of 1963. I just turned 22 years old. I must be the greatest."
- Muhammad Ali

If you *really* want something, believe me, you'll take action. You'll do whatever is necessary and you'll break through fears to get there.

I remember a millionaire I met once. He had always really wanted to be a millionaire. He told me that he read every book there was about millionaires. He did whatever those books said he should do - he did *exactly* what they said.

Every day, as he drove to work, he said out loud to himself "I am a millionaire". He'd repeat that statement thousands of times for the entire length of his hour-long journey. He did that every single day. That shows that he really wanted to be a millionaire. Really he did. He took action towards his dream. He did things other people read about but don't do. Now he is a millionaire.

Just like with me wanting to be Electra, I did so much every day in some way to make it a reality. I'd skate, sing, practise the part, work on my voice – I'd do whatever was necessary.

I really wanted to play Electra in Starlight.

Do you have a goal on your list that you're not achieving? If so, ask yourself the question: do I really want this goal? And if the answer is 'yes' ask yourself whether your fears are preventing you from taking the action you need to take to achieve that goal.

Many experts will tell you that the secret to goal setting and achievement is to let your mind run wild and free and to dream the big dreams. For me, that's fine up to a point but you'll end up writing things down that you think you should want and that you won't believe you could ever achieve.

I suggest you ask a different question – what do you want in your heart of hearts? What do you deeply desire?

What you really want could be very simple. For you, it might be to teach children. It might be to get out of debt. You'll know if it's what you really want because it will resonate with you just like wanting to play Electra in Starlight Express did for me. It will be something you can really identify with. Your heart will sing and you will feel excited.

YOU WILL GET WHAT YOU TRULY DESIRE

The Latin root meaning of the word desire is 'from the star'. If you really want something strongly enough – in other words if you truly desire rather than just want something – then the Universe will provide it to you. There's no guarantee on when or in what way, but it will happen. Of that there is no question.

So check in with your heart. It knows what you really want. Your head doesn't and most of the time we set goals that come from our head. We decide on what we want based on what society tells us that we should want. Or our ego gets in the way and tells us what we should have in order to look good in the eyes of others.

"One of the greatest discoveries a man makes, one of his great surprises, is to find he can do what he was afraid he couldn't do."
- Henry Ford, 1863-1947, Founder of Ford Motor Company.

So if there's something you really want to achieve, do or be, you'll come up against obstacles for sure. Plus you will feel fearful at some point but if you really want that thing you'll work through the problems.

And if you don't *really* want the goal –. in your heart, that is - when you meet obstacles or fear you won't take the action necessary to move closer to their realization.

YOU MUST IDENTIFY WITH AND RELATE TO YOUR GOALS

What's absolutely key is that you can relate to your goals. Can you truly identify with being, doing or achieving your goals? Can you see yourself having achieved them? If you can, then they will happen for you.

My friend Haddaway really identified with his goal of being a chart-topping singer. He lived a life worthy of a pop star before it ever happened for him. And the funny thing is that if you do this too then any fears you might feel aren't as powerful because in your mind you've already made it. Your enhanced identity allows you to break through the fears.

My identity is that I am a dancer, a choreographer, a coach, a trainer and I am a lover. I am strong and confident. I am passionate. I am energetic. I am a creator of abundance. I am rich. I am sexy. I am outrageous. I am funny. I am exciting. I am powerful. I am motivating. I am a leader. I am joyous. I am happy.

When I say those things my internal voice in my head does not say "no". There are no doubts. I do not hear the words "you are not" or "who are you kidding?" Actually, those words about who I am are not even coming from my head – they are coming from my heart.

In the past when I thought about money I'd sit there and not be able to get the identity of me being a millionaire into my body on a consistent basis. There's never been any congruency or passion there.

I used to want the things that society says you should want. When I suddenly gave up on that and decided to pursue the goals that I wanted it was such a relief.

And when you decide and go after the things that you really want the weird thing is that you wonder why you ever felt so scared in the first place. So my message to you is - do not worry.

So right now take a look at your list of goals if you have one. When you look at them check inside to see how they feel for you. If they don't resonate maybe they're the wrong goals for you.

I asked myself a question once – why do I want to become a millionaire? One reason that I came up with was that I wanted the prestige of being able to say that I was a millionaire. That felt right. I also thought I'd get respect through being a millionaire. And I realised that it was actually recognition I was seeking but that recognition could come to me without me having to make that kind of money.

And the more I thought about this issue the more I realised that what I really wanted about being a millionaire was to be free of the system. That's what I really want. Not being controlled by the system. So if income tax goes up by 1% I won't be bothered. If my mortgage payments rise by £300 a month, that won't faze me one bit. That's what I really want. That financial goal excites me and I can identify with that.

Money would give me freedom. Feeling free would mean doing just what I like. I would not have do things just for money.

Now I'm taking the actions that will lead towards me achieving financial freedom.

This whole concept of identity is very important. If you tell yourself that you are weak or a failure what actions do you then take? Ones that show weakness? Or failure? If you want to make changes in your life this concept is crucial to understand.

If a smoker stops smoking and you ask them, "Are you now a non-smoker?", often enough they cannot say yes with confidence, because being a non-smoker means just that. They do not smoke. Ever. They struggle with this because it is not yet their identity.

What happens if someone wants to lose weight but defines themself as a fat, overweight pig? How does someone with that identity live their life? To stay congruent with that identity they must do 'fat, piggish things'.

I coached someone once who was an alcoholic. He told me that during his therapy to get sober the therapist gave him a medicine that made him violently ill if he drank even a sip of alcohol. He still drank. I asked him why and he told me that he was an alcoholic and that's what alcoholics did. They drink. So he did. Even though doing so made him feel very unwell. He had to stay congruent with his identity.

Why do transsexuals go through such a drastic change of body just to have the body of the opposite sex? To them, it's their identity. **We do whatever it takes to stay congruent with our identity.**

So if there is something you want to become, you must identify with it. If you are fat and want to lose weight then you must identify with the body you want to have. If you smoke and want to stop you must identify yourself as a non-smoker. What do non-smokers do? They never smoke. You must identify yourself as a non-smoker at your core. If you do not then being a non-smoker will simply remain as a concept in your head.

THE 'GET A NEW IDENTITY' EXERCISE:

1. *What is your current identity? Come up with a list of all the ways – good and bad - that you currently define yourself as a person.*

2. *What do you really want in life – in your heart, what do you really want? Is to be a professional singer, to run a marathon, to be fit and healthy, to be a non-smoker, to be slim and attractive, to be a millionaire or to be a great father, mother, husband, wife or lover? Do a list. Keep going until there is nothing else you desire to come out.*

3. *Now, be honest - can you honestly in your heart, soul, core, bones, muscles and in every cell of your being identify with what you want to become? Really and truly? That is your next task. You need to start to walk the way that person you want to become would walk. You need to talk, eat, move, stand, breathe, act, react, respond and truly live like that person would. This is the key. It must become your identity. You must own this identity in your body. Make it yours every single day. Find a name you can call yourself – I am ..... Make this identity who you are from the inside and the actions will follow quite naturally. You need to do just what I did when I identified myself with playing the part of Electra and what Muhammad Ali did when he identified himself as being the greatest boxer of all time.*

Two other examples of this are that wonderful inspiring spirit, Madonna, and my friend Haddaway. Madonna told me a story about when she first went to New York. This was way before she became famous and she said to a taxi driver: "Remember my name because you'll be saying it one day." She was a complete unknown at the time but she had identified with being a star already.

Madonna and Haddaway lived their identities as stars before they had their hit records by the way they talked and acted and the people they associated with. So, in turn, the Universe just let them be who they were meant to be.

So whatever you want to be, find ways to live as that kind of person as often as possible. If you want to be a millionaire go to where they hang out and walk down expensive streets. Live and breathe as they do. See yourself in your mind's eye as the person you want to be. Think the same way that the people who have achieved what you want to achieve do. Act and be the person you want to become as often as possible. Learn your desired role in life like a choreographed routine. Have it become muscle memory.

I heard one of my role models, Denzel Washington, talking in an interview once saying that before doing a scene he taps his chest and says to himself: "Be honest, be honest. Don't act, just be honest". He becomes the character. For him, it's real. At that moment the role is his identity.

The powerful thing about identity is that even in times of uncertainty - because it is who you are - you will pull through because Nature insists that we stay congruent with our identity.

In show business we have the term 'the show must go on', meaning that no matter what happens you must deliver. And that's what amazing professional performers do – they deliver no matter what.

GET A CLEAR VISION

"The one without dreams is the one without wings."
Muhammad Ali

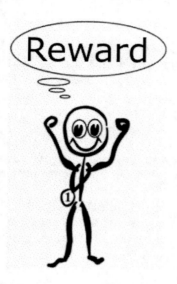

Vision is the ability to see. This means the ability to see what already exists with your eyes, but also to the ability to see what *could* exist in your *mind's* eye.

Your mind's eye is the place where all new creations begin. Everything that we can now see and use – from telephones, planes, computers, fitness centres, lights through to the wheel - all started out as a vision in someone's mind.

The powerful thing about having a vision is that you get pulled towards it. A vision has magnetic powers. The clearer the image, the stronger the power of attraction. The clearer and more precise the better.

Imagine you are driving your car on a foggy day and you are stuck in a car park. You want to get out but you cannot see where you are going. You drive hesitantly, feeling your way. Then the fog clears and you can see where you are going. You can see the exit so it's full steam ahead.

This story is a metaphor for how things are in terms of vision. If you don't have one you are uncertain. When you have one you can fly.

The vision can be big, small or grandiose - it doesn't matter. As long as you have one that resonates with you and you can believe you can achieve. That's all that matters. How you're going to get there isn't so important. But when you imagine your vision in your mind, you can connect with it emotionally. It makes you feel energized, empowered, excited and fulfilled. The more positive feelings you can associate with your vision, the better.

The subconscious mind does not know the difference between reality and perceived reality. For the subconscious mind whatever is envisioned will become real. This is why it is so important to 'police your mind' - if your visions and thoughts are mainly negative this will be what the subconscious mind will make real for you.

One way to police the mind is to consciously think positive thoughts and to feel things in a positive way. Affirmations are positive statements that you say to yourself about yourself or what you want to achieve. I believe that just doing affirmations isn't enough because you may not believe in what you're saying. I believe in stating affirmations with emotional intensity and moving your body to really feel and experience what you are saying. Own it. You should seek to create more and more muscle memory so that you truly identify with what you are saying.

Visualisation is a powerful technique whereby you consciously think, feel and experience in your mind and body what you want for your life. Doing this feeds your desires into your subconscious mind. It is important to engage all your senses in this process. What I mean by this is putting yourself completely in the scene that you want your life to be about. Seeing it as if you are the camera lens - seeing all the shapes and colours ... hearing all the sounds that going on around you ... hearing what other people are saying. Don't forget your senses of smell and touch either - so feel the wind or warm breeze ... touch the furnishings ... smell the atmosphere ... and feel the ground beneath your feet.

The more you can experience the vision in your body, the more real it becomes to your subconscious. The more you do this, the easier the technique becomes and the more you begin to own it in your nervous system.

The big lesson I learnt from my Electra experience was that:

... you have to have a crystal clear picture of exactly what you want

I saw myself in the part as often as possible. The feelings I got from just imagining being on stage, wearing the costume, hearing the audience and feeling the perspiration on my face were amazing. I had no clue at first as to how I was going to make it happen. There were lots of barriers but I didn't let them get in the way of my vision. Opportunities began to show up. Keep your vision alive and real and let the Universal laws do the rest.

Having a vision will give your life a true sense of meaning and purpose. You'll have something that compels you to act. You'll have more balance in your life and you'll be using your innate skills towards a positive outcome.

'VISUALIZATION' EXERCISE

Here's a visualization exercise:

1. *First, sit comfortably or lie down. Close your eyes and allow your thoughts to slow down. Eventually your thoughts will become 'alpha brainwaves' and you'll be able to feed your vision directly into your subconscious mind.*
2. *Take four deep breaths, breathing in through your nose and out through the mouth. Relax and let all the tension release from your body.*
3. *Then imagine your ideal world - you have more than enough money in the bank, you have lots of free time, you are free to pursue your passions, your desires. There are no limitations and no blocks and all you've ever wanted is now available to you. You are free to access it, obtain it, feel it and experience it.*
4. *Go with the flow - what do you imagine? What do you really want? What do you see? Feel the image surround you, growing and becoming more and more real each second. What can you hear? Who is there with you? What are they saying to you? How do you feel? What is the sense of inner power you have?*
5. *See it clearly. Feel it. Find a phrase and say it in your head to reinforce what this means to you. Feel, touch, smell and taste as much as possible.*
6. *Now see yourself making a commitment. See yourself with the power, the strength, the honour and the courage to put it into your body. Embed it in your being. Feed it to your core. Let it course through your veins. Fill your lungs with each breath you take. Move towards this. This is your vision.*

There is a saying that you can go through life like a leaf blown off a tree. It just blows around until it eventually lands on the ground. If it is lucky it'll land on the grass or something soft to take care of it. Or, if it's unlucky, it'll land on the road or in a puddle. Alternatively you can live your life like an arrow from a bow aimed at a target with laser-like focus. Which life do you choose?

CONGRUENCY

Some of the major influences and role models in my life have been people like Muhammad Ali, Malcolm X, Martin Luther King, the personal development guru Anthony Robbins, and Bruce Lee. These are people that, for me, are so congruent. Their actions match what they say.

When you watch them in action you notice that they communicate with their whole body and they generate an energy that inspires, heals, teaches, leads and motivates. Their passion is in the delivery of their words and they have a level of intensity that has you believing in them 100%.

Bruce Lee's physiology was completely congruent. As he spoke you could feel the intensity in his voice as well as his attention to detail. Also, when he trained his power, speed and agility were so amazing to watch. He was so disciplined that he trained everyday.

I look for this kind of congruency in people. If you examine great speakers from down the years – the likes of John F. Kennedy and Martin Luther King – you'll notice that it wasn't just their words that made an impact. It was how they delivered their message that upped the level of power they had to influence.

When you're congruent you can become a leader. When your physiology and your words are matched you have a presence. People gravitate towards you. They listen to what you have to say. They are inspired and strengthened by you.

I have discovered that I have the ability to uplift others. I didn't know I was doing it but, when I was in Starlight Express, people often said to me that when they were on stage with me they pushed themselves further. And I know that didn't happen just because of anything I said.

Words don't convince unless you walk your talk. Your credibility is your results. It's not that you've been through college because that proves nothing unless you go out into the real world and practise what you preach.

USE YOUR BODY

It's so easy to get 'stuck in a rut' but you can get out of it by using your body.

I've had coaching clients who'd come back week after week not having done the things we'd agreed upon the previous time we'd met. I'd be a little frustrated that they'd not moved forward and would, honestly, feel like physically shaking them.

And do you know what? Thinking back, if I had done that, it would have had a beneficial effect. By physically shaking them I would have got them out of their 'in a rut' state of mind.

Have you ever wondered why we have sayings in society such as 'pull yourself together' and 'shake yourself up'? It's because you don't just think yourself out of bad situations. You have to physically get yourself out of where you are so that you can move on.

My own experiences support this. As a dancer, physical movement and action are what I'm all about. When I'm not feeling ready to do what needs to be done with a dance routine, I physically shake myself out. That allows me to move in a different direction with my body.

IMPROVE YOUR SELF COMMUNICATION

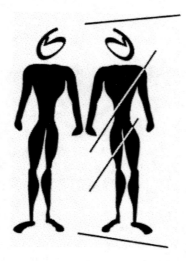

We are constantly communicating either with ourselves or to the outside world and, of course, we cannot communicate to the outside world before we've first communicated to ourselves.

There are three aspects to the way in which we communicate to ourselves. Together they determine the way we feel at any particular time. Psychologists refer to this as the self-communication triad.

The triad is the way we use our words, our body and our focus.

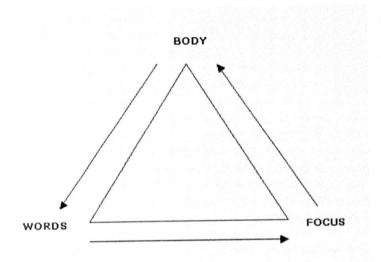

How these three aspects interact with each other determines how we feel and at what level.

Let's look at the body first of all. If I were to say to you that I, at this moment, was celebrating, you could tell me, I'm sure, what kind of things I was doing with my body. I had a big fat grin on my face, my arms were pumping in the air and I was jumping around the room. As a consequence I felt great. I didn't before I started but, because I did those things, I felt great.

Which goes to show that we actually *do* emotions. They don't only happen to us. If we use our bodies in certain ways, this allows us to access particular emotions, be they good or bad.

So let's say you wanted to feel confident - how would you use your body? How would you stand? Shoulders back? Chest out? Breathing deeply? What kind of tension would be in your muscles? You've surely felt confident before so remember back to how your body felt then.

Try this out as an experiment. Stand up and face the ceiling. Put a wide smile on your face, push your shoulders back and put your chest out and - without changing your physiology - attempt to feel sad.

You can't, can you? It's impossible to feel sad because this physiology triggers positive emotions in your body.

The words we use also have a significant impact on the way we feel and to what level. The scientific law of cause and effect states that if you do something, there will always be an effect. If you hit a nail with a hammer (cause) on a piece of wood then the effect will be the nail piercing the wood.

So too is the case with words. If you say a certain word (cause) you will get a result from what you have said (effect). For example, if you were to constantly use negative words such as terrible, grim, depressing, bad, gloom, doom, troubled, tragic, grieving, low spirits, long-faced, pessimistic, dreary, glum, forlorn and moping there's a pretty good chance you'd feel those feelings on a regular basis. In fact, I bet you felt disempowered as you read the words!

On the other hand, if you were to use words such as wonderful, amazing, brilliant, joyful, buzzing, sensational, fabulous, incredible, marvellous, exciting, blissful, great, excellent, energising, passionate, extraordinary, impressive and awesome then just imagine the effects that would be generated by the power of those words.

This is why it is important to choose your words carefully. Certain words send a powerful message to the subconscious and then to the cells, resulting in an effect in your body.

The next important aspect in self-communication is focus. What you focus on you will find. What you focus on seems real. What you focus on grows.

There is a wonderful saying from one of my great teachers, best-selling author Iyanla Vanzant: where the mind goes, the behind follows.

As a dancer I know the importance of having focus. When a dancer executes a succession of turns called pirouettes they do a unique movement with the head called 'spotting'. While the body is rotating the head of the dancer focuses on one point, that being the place they will move to after the end of the pirouette movements. So the dancer is turning but keeping their head looking at one spot - so the body is in effect turning without the head. Then, at the last minute, when the body can only turn so far without the head coming with it, the head is whipped back round to focus on the place where the body is intending to go.

This is done for three reasons:

- to make sure that the dancer doesn't get dizzy from pirouetting (some dancers can do 25 at a time)
- to be able to count the number of turns completed
- and, most importantly, so the dancer knows where they are going. The focus then directs the body to follow.

This is so key to life. We will only live for what we focus on. It is remarkable, but true.

Have you ever attempted to not think of something and in your attempt you are constantly thinking about the thing you are not meant to be thinking about? That's focus for you. Where the mind goes, the behind follows.

Is the glass half full or half empty? Do you look at the good or at the bad in a situation? To develop a successful lifestyle we must look at the good. We must focus on the good. How do we change our focus? The most powerful way to change our focus for the better is to ask a better question of yourself.

Examples of positive questions to ask are: How can I feel good right now? Is there something positive I can get out of this situation right now? Who do I love? Who is proud of me?

Successful people use this triad of words, focus and body to their advantage. They adopt a powerful physiology on a regular basis, they use positive self-talk and they focus on the good in every situation.

So going back to wanting to feel confident, I talked about what to do with your body. If you add to that positive self-talk - with you saying such things as "I feel strong and fantastic" - and focus back to a time from the past when you felt confident, you'll be using all aspects of the triad and you will feel amazingly confident.

Just as an actor learns his or her lines to a point that he or she can play their part without thinking, that is what you should strive for in terms of your stage – which is called your life.

It may take a little effort in the beginning but, as the body begins to learn, it will become second nature. So you could train yourself so that you feel confident most of the time. How powerful would that be?

GET ANCHORED

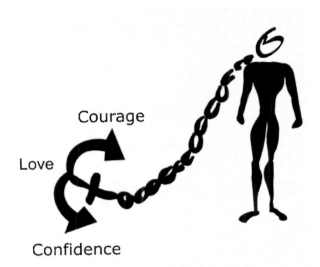

How powerful would it be to know that whenever you needed to be in a powerful, courageous, confident, excited, loving or proud emotional state for meetings, interviews, auditions, speaking engagements, negotiations or whatever, you could access these emotions in a fast and effective way?

The human body is amazing and is capable of so much. But wouldn't it be great if you could give it a signal that would automatically trigger you to go into a useful emotional state? Well, as far-fetched as it might seem, you can, thanks to a process known as anchoring.

This technique comes from the science known as Neuro-Linguistic Programming (NLP). With the technique you can condition your body to respond to a unique stimulus in a positive way without any conscious effort on your part.

For an anchor to be created the body must be in an intense emotional state. Then something unique has to happen, either visually, audibly or kinaesthetically (touch or feeling). This trigger or stimulus must occur often during this peak emotional experience as this will be the key for it to be locked into the body. The more times the unique stimulus is executed during the peak emotional state, the stronger the anchor will be.

Anchors are nothing new. It's just that the process of anchoring has only recently been identified, given a name and mastered.

Many anchors get created within people on a daily basis without them even being aware. Many others are formed via the media and advertising. Commercials are normally repeated time and time again and if people are in a positive emotional state whilst watching or listening to them, then they'll find that they end up with a strong anchor to the product. And before they know it at 11.30 in the office they'll unwittingly find themselves reaching for a certain brand of diet cola, for example!

Whenever a person is in an intense emotional state in which the whole body and mind are involved and something unique consistently happens to the body, a neurological link from the brain to the emotion is formed. Whatever the unique link is will automatically trigger the person to go back to that emotional state.

When you think back, there will be certain songs that when you hear them on the radio remind you of a certain time and place. The emotions, be they positive or negative, that you felt back then will come back to you. That song is an anchor.

Other examples are great speeches from great leaders and national anthems. Strong emotions are normally stirred when you first hear them and you'll find that, hearing the words or music again, will bring back those original emotions within you.

When you smell again a particular perfume or aftershave that a special ex-partner used to wear memories of when you were with them will come flooding back. That smell is an anchor.

In fact, smells are particularly powerful anchors. This dates back to our ancient roots when the sense of smell was crucial to survival. Man needed high sensitivity to smells because that is how they would anticipate the arrival of prey or a predator and prepare themselves to take the necessary action.

Anchors can be negative as well as positive. Think what emotions, memories and reactions the sight of a Nazi swastika or a burning cross evokes in people.

The way to go with this is to take control and to use anchors in a way that can benefit us. This means to consciously set up our own positive anchors.

The keys to setting up anchors successfully are:

1. Choose a trigger that is unique – for example, a mannerism that you do not do regularly such as touching one of your ear lobes with the little finger of your opposite hand or pulling a finger in a certain way. A hand clap or snapping your fingers are not unique enough.

2. Put yourself into the emotional state you want to trigger by experiencing vividly a time from your past when you were in this state.

3. Pick an experience that is pure and not mixed with other feelings.

4. Timing is crucial, so fire the anchor at the peak of the experience and release before the peak declines.

5. Spend time at anchoring to become skilful. The more times the anchor is fired at the peak of the experience, the stronger the anchor will become.

6. Once the anchor has been established, whenever you want to experience this particular emotion, you simply need to activate the trigger exactly as it was applied in order to relive the emotional state.

Imagine being able go onto stage, walk into a business meeting, enter important negotiations or attend a job interview or an audition and being able fire off a 'confidence or courageous anchor' that immediately puts you into that emotional state that makes you resourceful enough to produce the success that you want.

USE YOUR CORE ENERGY

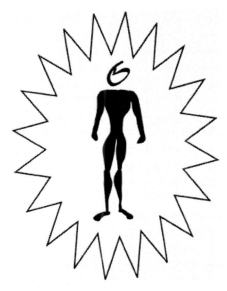

"Let a woman be a woman and a man be a man."
- Prince

Your body is your home on Earth, so think for a moment about the harmonious way in which it supports you in your life.

Think about the finest of adjustments it makes to coordinate your muscles, skeleton, blood, skin, arteries, veins and organs. Notice how it all works together so rhythmically to function and take you forward in life. Think about how the strength and support of your legs and back allow you to stand upright. Consider the movement involved in running, jumping, sitting, lying, standing, climbing, bending, spinning and tumbling. It all happens in complete trust and harmony as we achieve the things in life we pursue.

We have a remarkable energy within us that creates and generates movements. This energy is something we are to evolve as we continue through our journey in life. We embody so many gifts within our structure as well as conscious thought, emotions and the ability to create new life. When we realise this energy, we understand that we are responsible for our life and can therefore participate in its success, healing and direction.

Think how remarkable the simple act of walking is. Pushing out one foot and the power going through each joint and through into the ground ... the contraction of the right muscles ... the bending of the knee ... the movement of the hips ... the swing of the arms - everything working so harmoniously together to propel you forward.

Think about how a woman's body transforms to become the vessel for motherhood. Notice how it changes to carry a child during pregnancy and how the body tunes in exactly in order to provide the right nutrients to the baby at the right time.

Think about the creative flow of energy within artists, designers, dancers, singers, songwriters and composers. Consider how their bodies adjust to produce the results they want. Think about athletes and how disciplined they are to train to get into shape to perform at their absolute peak of fitness.

It is magnificent when this flow of energy is used to create health, love and success. This energy has the power to heal and to generate what we are and want in life.

This energy takes us to the understanding that we can be responsible for our own healing. Our internal power is waiting for the bio-chemical messages to be sent by our subconscious mind. Once we are aware of this we can move, breathe and act differently as regarding taking responsible steps towards our own healing. This is a fantastic example of how the body works beautifully in harmony with itself.

In my early dancing career I always had lotions, creams, medications and painkillers with me so that I could survive each show I was doing. Since I became aware of this energy, I have come to realise the effects of positive energy and how I am responsible for how I feel and how I heal. Because I now take care of my body in healthy and positive ways using this energy, I haven't taken any medication for years. I also feel that I have more energy than I did ten years ago.

The power to move with grace, skill, strength and co-ordination is a masterful display of the internal energy our bodies possess.

We've heard the story about the child being trapped under a car and the mother finding the super-human strength to lift the car to free the child. This shows how focused our energy can become to deliver the results we really want.

We are aware of the potency and power of sexual energy. It is nature's way of ensuring the survival of the species by creating a strong intimate bond between two people. It creates life. It creates pleasure and joy, as well as self-exploration and expression. It takes you to places in yourself that ignite deeper levels of sensuality and consciousness. Sex is a beautiful and natural act, which must be entered into without guilt or shame. During uninhibited sex you are completely living in the moment, a time when all fears and anxieties disappear and you become one with the flow of life itself.

Within dance we witness and experience the movement of the hips and pelvic area through rotation, thrusting and gyrating. The potent sexual energy that is generated by these movements is so strong and hypnotic that they, of themselves, will generate a truly intimate bond. The combined sexual energy that can be formed when two people dance together can be so beautifully intoxicating as their energies interlink.

Have you noticed the way that most women dance? They generally move and rotate their hips, instinctively putting out a signal to entice their mate to connect with this energy.

Many men are much more limited in their movement of the hips. This is because they believe that it is not very masculine to move this area of the body freely. I find that this energy has often been suppressed for so long that there is a block in the energy flow within the body. When men are freer in this area they connect fully to the energy.

The hips and lower abdomen area are the power centre of the human body as it is from here that we become centred and grounded. This area generates the most energy for us to move successfully. So much in life can take us off balance and the energy generated here aids inner calm and strength.

In my movement workshops, I work a lot on these areas. My aim is to loosen and create more freedom and co-ordination in the hip and pelvic areas and to strengthen the abdomen and lower back muscles to allow maximum flow from the centre.

I have realised and discovered through my spirit that I am moving and striving for balance. My intentions, teachings and learning along my journey are all moving me towards a balanced life. There is a natural energy that has to be in balance.

There is positive and negative, black and white, yin and yang and masculine and feminine. In our beings we have these energies but often they are out of balance. With Nature's need to maintain balance these energies naturally seek out their opposite.

We are men and women who have a need for each other in an interdependent way for our survival and reproduction. We are constantly evolving, and within us evolve these energies. Masculine and feminine energy are in us all, but through conditioning, lifestyle and learning one tends to dominate the other, in our need for survival in our particular environment, culture or community.

The attraction and interdependence of the human race depend on these masculine and feminine energies and act like a magnet of attraction to their opposites.

As a man or woman, you will possess both masculine and feminine energies but one of these energies may dominate you at the core of who you are. A man with feminine energy at his core will tend to be softer, more tender and compassionate. Whereas a man with masculine energy at his core will tend to be a strong decision maker, will take action and will have the power to really focus.

A woman who is feminine at the core of her being will tend to be freer, tender, softer and will emanate femininity.

Within the natural laws of the Universe there is a natural attraction to opposites. A man strong in masculine energy will tend to be attracted to a woman strong in feminine. A woman with masculine energy will tend to be attracted to a man with feminine energy.

Remember we are talking about energy - the energy that is dominant at the core of your being. This does not mean that you cannot and do not have access to the opposite energy within you. A man with masculine energy at his core can also be tender, compassionate, caring and free. Equally a woman with feminine energy can make decisions and has the power to focus and take control of a situation.

Here are some examples of the differences between the energies.

Masculine Energy	Feminine Energy
Tends to reach outward	Tends to reach inward
Deals with outer world	Deals with inner world
Generalises	More detailed
Intellect, thought, logic	More from emotion
More aggressive	More compassionate
More focused thinking	More free thinking
About releasing	About filling up
Conscious mind	Subconscious mind
From the head	From the heart
Making big things small	Making small things big
Hard and direct	Soft and flexible

The aim in Nature is to move you towards becoming balanced in yourself so you will therefore attract someone who can put balance in your life.

For example, I am masculine at my core. Through my profession, learning and self-discovery I have developed and utilise the feminine energy within me. This growing in my being allows me to access both energies often which means I will be attracted to a woman feminine at her core but with some balance similar to my own.

The balance is about making and taking decisions based on what feels right, rather than what seems to be just the logical thing to do. Men may not want to admit it, but they are more often ruled by the hearts and not by their heads.

Within the Universe energy in balance is clearly seen and displayed through the interactions and balance of the sun and the moon. Our world depends on the interdependence of these two bodies. The sun is like masculine energy and tends to stand out and be bold whereas the moon calmly does its thing at night and has a profound effect on the mood of the planet.

These masculine and feminine energies show up in the way we use our bodies. Men can be stopped in their tracks by watching a woman walk into a room and swoon because of her ability to emanate feminine energy. Also a man oozing masculine energy will cause many women to go weak at the knees.

The physical manifestation of these energies lies in the different ways in which men and women stand, walk, talk, hold their posture, carry out gestures, make eye contact, move their hands and legs and so on.

Many people underestimate the power of this energy. In job interviews, castings and auditions judgements are made as you enter a room. So what is your energy saying?

In some of my movement workshops I do an exercise to do with walking. The way you walk speaks for the kind of person you are or want to be. Most people aren't aware of the energy and messages they put out by the way they walk. I'm referring to the way they hold themselves, how they use or swing their arms, whether they have their shoulders back, whether their chest is out or collapsed, does their head do a chicken nod as they walk and so on.

When I work with actors it is interesting to watch them perfect the walk of the character that they are to play. You can literally see them take on the physical characteristics of a personality through their walk.

Have you ever noticed when an actor is portraying a gangster? Have you noticed the way they walk? How they enter a room? Robert De Niro is a classic example as he literally owns the whole room by virtue of the way he walks as a gangster.

If you want to look like success, how about walking for success? Does your walk signify complete confidence? Courage? Ease? Flexibility? Strength? Joy? Love? Happiness? Failure? Weakness? Shyness? Timidity? Honour? Your walk portrays the energy that you are most often using from within your being.

The way we use our bodies is so key to what we want to achieve in life. It is a very powerful gift we have. Think clearly of the message that you want to give out.

I once did a TV pilot for a self-development programme where I had to coach a man on dating. His challenge was that girls always thought he was a great and dear friend but not someone they would date or want to date.

With a few questions I discovered that he was, in fact, masculine at the core of his being but somehow could not access that aspect of him when it came to interacting with women. I asked him what kind of things he talked about when he met a woman. He said that he discussed her hairstyle and clothes, which shops she bought from and so on. In short, the kind of things a good friend would talk about. Remember the list of masculine and feminine energies? Remember that the feminine energy will tend to make small things big? "Nice coat, where did you get it from? I love what you've done with your hair," is an example of the feminine energy talking.

So we did some movements to get him in touch with his true core of masculine energy and we tested this new energy out on a woman. After a few minutes I explained to her what I had done and asked her about his new approach to her.

She said that he came across as confident and seemed to know what he wanted. She said that she liked that in a man. This was a fantastic display of how using your body differently can give you different results.

With these energies, women can often fall into the biggest trap. Women need to take care because as they get older and take on more responsibilities in business and at home they can lose touch with their feminine core and take on more masculine energies. The danger with this situation is that they will become less attractive to a man with masculine energy at his core.

So if they have a masculine husband or partner there will be a loss of attraction. He may begin to be attracted to a woman with more feminine energies – the classic 'husband leaving wife of 30 years for the 20 year old secretary' syndrome.

Men are a little luckier in the sense that the older they get, the more masculine they may become by virtue of what they do at business and in the home - hence the 20 year old girl's attraction to the older man!

The key for women is to keep the balance. Women need to keep in touch with their feminine energies allowing themselves to be all the woman they are. Look at some great women like Goldie Hawn, Sophia Loren and Oprah Winfrey and how they have kept in touch with their free-spirited feminine side whilst becoming astute businesswomen.

Again, the most important thing for men and women to strive for is balance. If men were to access and be more in touch with their feminine energies, there would be fewer wars, rapes, acts of abuse and violence and greed in the world.

In fact, this whole issue is the essence of my show 'The Vital Fire'. It is based on the spiritual journey of the growth of a man. He re-evaluates love, war and work and uses the power within himself by being in touch with his feminine energy.

This is how I feel the new man is evolving. No longer are many men only about suppressing emotions and being this violent soldier that feels nothing and denies compassion and empathy. Many are freeing themselves to simply enjoy the nature of all things and the simplicity of life itself.

This is demonstrated through acrobatics, dance and song as the story follows the man on his own journey towards balance. He confronts the warrior and money-crazed businessman and discovers how becoming more balanced enables him to have the power and ability to influence a whole nation.

MOVE WITH PASSION

You can really see the difference in results between the professionals and amateurs. Take singing. As an example, Celine Dion has incredible natural talent but still constantly strives to do better and to work at her craft. All these years on she still does her one hour warm up every day and often doesn't speak for two days before any performance. She respects and honours her gift.

Passion is a key in all of this. It gives you the energy. It's an emotion that some people rarely experience. They go to a job they hate, come home and deal with regular things but never do anything with any kind of enthusiasm.

The job you do may not be your ideal job but you can find passion in most places. You can find some sort of intensity and some pleasure in almost anything you do.

If you experience passion in your life you'll have a great time. You'll feel it when you want something so badly. You'll have the determination and commitment to make things happen in spite of fear, limitations and blocks.

Passion means everything. You should strive to connect with your partner, children, your job and your friends in a truly passionate way. If you do, joy will be never-ending and everything you experience in life will feel new and exciting.

I recently met up again with an ex-girlfriend of mine. We had such a passionate relationship and when I looked into her eyes and saw that passion again, I told her that was what kept me attracted to her.

I really relate to passion in any field. I love versatility and when I see someone with passion I am entranced by them. It triggers something inside me. I feel that I've connected with a similar soul and kindred spirit.

When people are passionate about something they become animated and their eyes light up. Watch a great actor being interviewed about great parts they've played and notice them ignite and light up inside their being. That kind of passion and enthusiasm is life to me. It's what life is all about.

When you see someone who doesn't enjoy what they're doing there is a dullness. There is no spark to what they're doing. I love to see fire.

Life is about expressing to everyone who you are. So often life isn't about the things we spend most of our time doing.

You can be out there trying to make lots of money and acquire possessions, but life itself isn't those things. It's about what you can feel, what you can express and what you are sensitive to. That's where the fire is. It's living passionately rather than pursuing all the time.

I saw George Best being interviewed on TV a few years ago. He said that he still relives the days when he was scoring goals in front of 50,000 people. He said that, since he retired, he's found it really difficult replacing those highs. That was what he was good at and his career was so short-lived.

MOTIVATION IS WHAT WILL GET YOU MOVING

**Until one is committed there is always hesitancy,
The chance to draw back, always ineffectiveness.
The moment one definitely commits oneself, then
providence moves too.
All sorts of things occur to help that would never
otherwise have occurred.
A whole stream of events issues from the decision, raising
to one's favour all manner of unforeseen accidents and
meetings and material assistance which no man could
have dreamed would come his way.
Whatever you can do or dream you can, begin it.
Boldness has genius, power and magic in it.
- Johann Wolfgang von Goethe**

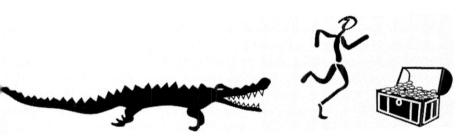

H ere are a couple of stories.

Story 1

"The first thing I do when I get up in the morning is to drink some water. Then I get dressed and do some deep breathing. Then I go for a run for about an hour. I come back and take a shower.

I go to work and afterwards I go to the gym. I jump rope for about 60 minutes, do 1,000 sit ups, push some weights and then I have a nice long stretch out of my muscles. Then maybe I take a class, if there is something I want to do, like yoga, Pilates or dance.

It feels fantastic. It pays to train. I know that I always want to feel great and full of energy, vitality, strength and power. I want my body to stay ripped and well defined with lean muscle. I know that when I'm in my 80s and 90s that I want to feel great and alive. I want to always strive to be better, stronger, wiser, healthier, fitter. I want to always feel the zest for life and all it has to offer. I want to generate energy, joy and happiness. I want to live a life of passionate moments. I want to strive to be a better person and to be around better people.

Just knowing what I want spurs me on daily to keep on living and charging my energy every day possible.

Story 2

After I struggle to get out of bed in the morning, I take a shower and get dressed. I have some coffee and toast, pack my things, just about get my child off to school on time and then head to work.

I come home and think about whether or not I should go to the gym later in the evening or sit down in front of the TV and order a Chinese takeaway. I think to myself, "If I don't do something about my weight soon I'll start getting problems that I don't want. I actually don't want to get fat. I know that I don't want people to look at me when I pick up my child from school and to think of me as fat." I don't want to have to avoid looking at myself in mirrors and I don't want the feeling of being out of breath when walking up a few stairs. I don't want to get older and slower. I don't want the feeling of heaviness and no energy.

Although I love my comforts and little vices, I know that I don't want to have the feeling that I could have prevented feeling slow and low on energy.

I know it's the way I am. If something doesn't come along and literally wake me up to the things that I may suffer with later on in life then I know that I'll just sit back with my creature comforts."

Two interesting stories and two very different reasons for taking care of the issue of health. Two different motives. Two different reasons to produce motion or action. It is what induces a person to act that is their motivation.

As we all know, humans are not random creatures. Everything we do is for a reason. Motivation plays a huge part in what we do or do not do. Motivation can be explained as the intensity and direction of a person's effort to a particular thing.

Many factors can play a part in an individual's reasons to be motivated. Several factors will be internal and several external. It is fascinating to observe how people are motivated, as people often act out their own views of motivation, consciously as well as subconsciously.

Although there may seem to be thousands of ways to be motivated there are actually only two main types – internal motivation, which is when the desire comes from within you, and external motivation, which is when the stimulus comes from outside of you.

What's interesting is that we all do want something, we all do want to feel better and we all do want a better life. But what is our motivation strategy to get what we want? What will it take for us to take the necessary action? What will be our motive?

Looking at our two stories again, we can clearly notice that the first person is motivated by what they want. This person is clear about how they want to feel in the future. This generates a drive to keep motivated.

The second person is clearly motivated by what they don't want. Only the thought of the pain or suffering that they may endure because of not taking action provides the incentive and motivation to move from where they are.

It is important that you know your motivation strategy. If you are to gain success in your life in any area, it is important to know your own motivation strategy. There isn't a right or wrong way to be motivated - there is only your way.

Think about times from your past when you were motivated to do something. Was your motivation based on wanting or not wanting something? Or was it both? Think about it carefully.

Coaches and therapists seek to find this out and use the information to help bring about positive change for their clients.

I know that I am motivated by what I want, what I can gain and what benefits I will obtain by certain actions. I am very definitely a 'move towards' person. A good friend of mine will only move if he has to, meaning his motivation will only be activated if he knows what he will lose or miss out on.

If you tell me what I will miss out on it will not be a strong enough motivator for me. This really isn't my way to be motivated. If I tell my friend all the great things and benefits he will get from taking action it will not motivate him in any way.

Once you have this information about yourself or someone else, small and subtle changes to how you express something will switch their or your own level of motivation.

An implication of this is that 'moving towards' people tend to be attracted to new possibilities whereas 'moving away from' people tend to act out of a sense of necessity. They will think about what it will cost them if they do not take action - but also they may only take the action when the costs or suffering are actually right there in front of them. So they get up and move because they have to.

You may notice this with smokers and people who are overweight. They know what it will cost them in life to continue living that way, but they will only stop when it is absolutely necessary. It may take the need to have an operation to have a nicotine-poisoned leg removed or a heart attack to get them to stop.

There are 26 billion cigarettes smoked every day so it is clear that millions of people have a 'moving away from' motivation strategy that only kicks in out of necessity.

There's a wonderful story about a woman who at one time weighed over 400kgs (860lbs) but thanks to years of motivation managed to lose over 280kgs (616lbs). I will keep her details anonymous, but hers is a quite amazing story that just has to be told.

As a young girl she was sexually abused, and as a result began eating and eating for her comfort and protection. She didn't want to look attractive to the opposite sex to prevent something like that ever happening again.

She said she would eat until the pain of the experience began to stop. She knew she was running away from those feelings and she used anger and resentment to cover up her pain. Before she knew it her weight was ballooning over 250kgs (550lbs).

When she was warned by her doctor to do something drastic or suffer serious consequences, she was up to 380kgs (836lbs). She could no longer breathe and she began to drown in her own fluids. Her skin began tearing because it had been stretched to its limit.

Incredibly, she kept on eating because it was her only joy and comfort in life. When she was eventually rushed to the hospital (in a kind of fork lift truck) she weighed over 400kgs.

The doctors thought that this was really the end of the road for her. She overheard them telling the staff to simply take care of her for her last few days.

While lying there in a reinforced constructed bed she knew that she had to do something. She didn't want to give her power away any longer as she had been doing all her life. Now she was about to die because of it and she said no. She knew that she had been angry and resentful all her life. She realised that this incident was robbing her of any life she had left. She said to herself, "no more."

This gave her the drive to do something. She now had the courage and determination to make a change. She was no longer the little girl that needed all that protection. She realised that she was a strong and powerful being and had the power to change her situation.

From then on she began to exercise. This meant just moving and walking at first. She learned about nutrition and realised why she was eating.

She didn't want to give away her power to the past any more. Over the next 8 years she lost over 280kgs!

In a way, she was grateful for having the near death experience. That woke her up into realizing that she had been holding onto the past.

For her it now feels great to be able to run, tie her own shoelaces, take a regular bath, pick up things from the floor. In other words, things that most people take for granted in terms of being able to do, she feels grateful for now being able to do.

For years she couldn't look at herself in the mirror but now she looks at herself and says "thank you" to her body - the body with which she can now feel and express happiness, joy, and pride. She now has the energy to enjoy more of life's pleasures again.

What is her motivation strategy?
Move away from or towards? Possibility or necessity?

I remember having dance teachers who would try to motivate us pupils with the costs of not working hard during lessons. They would say things like, "you will never make it in this profession if you don't work harder. No-one will hire you." I would always say to myself, "yes they will. There is always another class I can go to where they appreciate my talents".

The teachers that I got along with the best were the ones that were encouraging. They would show me the rewards of hard work and would tell me that opportunities would arise and that all the doors would open if I could execute and learn certain things. That inspired me and moved me to the maximum.

Again, no teacher was right or wrong, but the moving towards is clearly the way for me. Tell me the rewards I'll get, and I'm motivated. Tell others what they will suffer if they don't move and that will work for them as far as motivation is concerned.

The key thing to keeping your motivation alive is to feed the motivation. Once you discover what internally motivates you, it is important to use that as often as possible and to remind yourself of that in many ways.

If you are a 'move towards' person, then remind yourself of, or visualise, the rewards and benefits that you will get by taking action.

If you are a 'moving away from' person then remind yourself of the things you will lose and miss out on and use these facts to keep you striving.

As motivation is the intensity and direction of your efforts it is important to commit to actions that will enhance your motivation.

External means of motivation may include telling others or sharing what you intend to do so that they hold you to it. Manipulate your environment to help your motivation. Join a group or community that makes you committed to follow through with your actions.

Sometimes the need to impress will keep your motivation alive. Other people are motivated by competition or by being really aware of the feelings that they will get if they achieve their goal. Again, having the ability to really identify with what you want to achieve will allow you to access those feelings and will enhance your motivation.

One of the best motivators is love. Loving what you are doing or pursuing is very powerful. If you experience love then you are motivated for the right reasons. To give love, receive love and experience love while taking action will make it all worthwhile.

This is what motivates me. If I can experience love for myself and others, then that will move me. It is a strong driving force, something that I use with clients also. I always start with love in all that I'm pursuing. I look for love always. I must love what I'm doing, love the results I'm pursuing and love myself for taking action.

I love to touch and inspire others by my actions and want to be a motivation to others by the actions I take and lifestyle that I live. My lifestyle has come about through love and pursuit of love. It is a strong motivator.

Use love in as many ways as you can in life. I see so many people just going through the motions in life, their work and their recreation. If they could only find love in what they were doing or wanting to do, it would make all the difference to their world.

The real success of motivation is to do with the feelings you will experience because of your achievement. These feelings you can already use to your advantage, because the feelings you are pursuing you already have and know. They can be the energy that you work with in pursuit of your success.

If you want happiness, joy, passion, love then access those feelings as often as possible through imagination and visualisation. Allow your body to experience the feelings you want so that you will then attract more of this energy towards yourself. Let that be a great motivator to gain even more of those feelings.

Another strong key to increasing your motivation is commitment. Making a commitment to do something is powerful. A true commitment that you will deliver to yourself or to someone or something external will give you a sense that there is no turning back. Just like a parachute jumper; once they have jumped there is no turning back.

True commitment is going where you want to go and knowing that there is no turning back. This will motivate you to deliver. You have made a decision, something that you are truly committed to. True commitment is something internal. It is a bond of integrity and honour. It is a standard that you set for yourself to hold to your word.

If someone becomes a parent then they are making a true commitment to being a father or mother - there is no turning back. A parent can also decide that they want a great and loving relationship with their children. This means making an internal commitment to being a good, loving, caring and compassionate mother or father.

Commitment is a bond you have with yourself that gives you the motivation to deliver and then be successful with what you want to achieve. Remember, everything we want to achieve on the outside starts with achieving it on the inside first.

In the movie 'Rob Roy', Liam Neeson's character has to duel with one of the finest swordsmen in England. He makes a commitment to his wife that he will return. He gives her his word. His bond. His commitment. Just making that commitment to himself and to his wife gives him the motivation to do whatever it takes to make sure he holds true to his word and his honour.

Another key motivator is to know specifically what it is you want to be a success at and to know how your success will benefit and serve others. The need for selfish success will not be success for the long term. However, by knowing that your success will be of service to others in some way you can be sure it will be true and lasting.

If you want a great and happy relationship, to attain your ideal weight, run your own business, become a great actor or become a millionaire, check that your intentions are to be of benefit to others through inspiration, love, contribution, sharing, caring, bonding and so on.

The great Nelson Mandela was motivated to keep going in spite of over 25 years of imprisonment because he knew his life was of great service to his people, his country and the world. He was motivated into preparing to run his country and setting the people free.

Like everything else to do with the body, motivation is a muscle that needs to be worked in order for it to work the way that you want. You can - like in a gym working physical muscles - start to train with smaller weights. Build the strength of your motivation muscle gradually. When you start to see and experience success, then you can up the weights to which you subject your motivation muscles.

Motivation separates the walkers from the talkers. If you haven't walked your talk it's because you were not motivated enough to do so.

We all have experienced times with ourselves or with others when something has been said and then should have been done but wasn't. It all comes down to motives. How important is it to deliver? How important is the outcome? Do you really want it? Really?

We all know the saying, "Actions speak louder than words." Well it is as simple as that. Do not go by what someone says but go by what they do. When people say "I love you", remember that love, as well as being a feeling, is also a verb. It is a doing word, an action. Loving actions have the intention of creating a loving environment or partnership.

Again, knowing what you want to achieve specifically is crucial to motivation, because if you are not sure of what you want then the motivation lessens or becomes sporadic. You lose focus and the motivation is not sustainable. Know specifically the success you want to experience.

So once you have clarity about the success you want and how to motivate yourself, it is then up to you to make the actions happen.

It is now time to put all of this into your body. Just knowing this material intellectually is not enough. Feel it. Pass it from your head to your whole body. Feel it resonate through to your inner core. Own it. Be it. Commit it to your muscles and bones. Put the feeling of commitment to your very soul. Honour your success with the commitment of love, determination, courage and truth. Feel the very thing you want deep in your heart. Let your cells be alive, focused, energised and working at achieving the very thing that your whole being wants. Know this to be the truth for you.

I have had the most success in my life because of this. Things or situations that I wanted happened because of living and breathing the outcome that I wanted. This has always been a great motivator for me.

HONOUR YOUR BODY

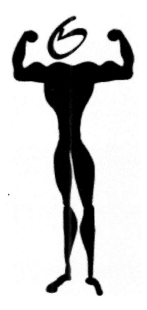

Your body is remarkable. It is your home on Earth. It will express all your emotions and creativity and will absorb all the information and knowledge you provide for it. It will take on all the symptoms and warning signals when things are out of balance and will let you know when your personality and life's purpose are aligned.

Whatever you feed it - emotionally, physically or psychologically - will become part of your being. Each part of the human body holds onto the memories of its experiences. Your cells get conditioned and programmed to the signals they are fed; that's why it's so important to use your body in ways that are positive.

The body rarely tells lies. Our mind can play tricks on us. We have thousands of thoughts and we can change our minds often.

The body, however, gives us clear signals - called intuition, instinct or the sixth sense - if we care to notice them. When we are stressed, exhausted, ill or suffering from disease, these are all signs from our body that we are out of balance in some way.

Babies know best and are in tune with their bodies. Notice the way a baby learns to express itself. First, it does it through eye contact only. Then it learns that it can communicate with head, arm and leg movements. Slowly babies discover smiling and use it to emanate pure love. Soon a baby will discover how to express itself through moving its body and, as the years go by, it expresses through laughter, jumping around and running. A baby enjoys life and all its riches.

Soon enough, boundaries are set for safety reasons and adults begin to suppress certain levels of emotion in the child. Then the child may disconnect from many forms of emotional expression. After that, academic learning takes over and certain creative, expressive, emotional outlets – such as dancing, singing, playing and sports - can end up being pushed down and even lost.

Be that as it may, you're an adult now and you are where you are. You can rectify a bad current situation with your body. And taking care of your body not only means that you have more fun, energy and vitality, but it also raises your chances of living a disease-free life.

Just one look at the statistics tells us how important it is to do all we can to avoid a hastened death or spending the last years of our life in pain:

- 1 in 4 men will have a heart attack before they reach the age of 65
- 1 in 3 people are developing some form of cancer

- 8 out of 10 people will suffer from some form of arthritis

Nevertheless, scientists have proven we have the capabilities to live a healthy life up to 100 years old.

There are a few keys and this is not rocket science. What I'll advise you to do is also pretty easy to implement in your life.

OXYGEN

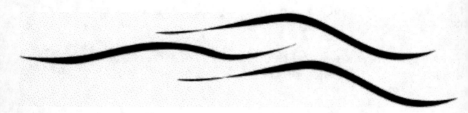

The most important fuel for the body is oxygen. It is the source of all life and without it everything dies.

Breathing in oxygen is something that most people don't think about. It simply happens without any kind of conscious thought, so people don't realize that they can do a lot to improve the way they breathe which, in turn, will improve their health.

Oxygen is our life energy and carries a bio-electric charge, called in Eastern civilisations either Chi, Ki, or Prana. Western science has established that the building blocks of the human body – cells - will always survive so long as they are surrounded by oxygen, and have the right nutrients.

Whenever I do any personal training or workshops the first thing I do is to work with the breath. Why this is so important is that, in times of stress or tension, we often deprive ourselves of deep breaths.

These days, with our busy lifestyles, we spend most of the time breathing shallowly and running our brain in 'betawave' state. This way of living contributes to illness and disease and robs us of energy.

So what most people do is to pump 'quick-fix' sources of energy into their body such as confectionery and coffee. This lifestyle forces the body to run on adrenaline and cortisol, which is highly toxic for the body. Adrenaline is only intended for use in emergencies so using it more often puts a great strain on the body's systems, again robbing you of energy and contributing to illness and disease.

Deep breathing:

- completely re-energises the body
- increases blood circulation
- boosts the immune system
- feeds the brain with more oxygen, which improves concentration levels and focus
- has a calming influence
- stops the body from over-stressing the adrenal glands
- aids sleep

It also has a very alkalizing effect that neutralizes the damaging acid build-up that is created in our bodies. The acidity many people suffer from is caused by a destructive lifestyle made up of too much stress, poor nutrition, too many negative emotions and physical strain. Oxygen's molecular structure includes a negative ion and its electrical charge is alkalizing. There is something called the PH scale, which measures the levels of acid and alkaline in a substance. This scale goes from 1-14, where 1-7 is measured as being acidic and 7-14 as being alkaline. Our blood functions in an alkaline environment.

Deep breathing also activates the lymph in our blood, which is responsible for immunity and cleansing our systems of toxins. Lymph is not pumped around the body automatically and is only activated by deep breathing or physical movement.

Deep breathing increases the level of lymph system activity by up to 15 times. So deep breathing can dramatically improve your capacity to fight off illness.

Breathing is in fact the only vital body function that is voluntary as well as involuntary. In other words, it will occur if you don't think about it but you can take conscious charge and breathe in a different way for a while.

This means we can have a link from the conscious to the unconscious. Notice also that breathing is a large part of disciplines such as meditation, yoga and the martial arts, all of which call on working out the body from the inside.

Every thought, movement and emotion manifests itself in the way you breathe. When you are fearful or nervous, for example, your breath is shallow and fast, whereas if you are calm and at peace your breath is slow and deep. So if you are nervous and consciously slow down your breath, you will calm down.

Deep breathing involves taking air into your more spacious lower lungs. You do this by pushing your stomach outwards as you breathe in and pushing your stomach in as you breathe out. This allows your lungs to fill up completely. You should not lift your shoulders and chest as this shuts out the lower lungs.

If you're not sure how this is done watch a baby when it is sleeping and you will notice its tiny stomach go in and out.

You can practise this technique by lying on the floor with a book on your chest. Deep breathe by pushing your stomach in and out and making sure that the book doesn't move.

It takes a little practice. Once mastered, eventually this way of breathing will become your natural state as it is mine. The benefits will be that you will become calmer, better able to concentrate, will sleep better, will be more energized and will have an alkalized system.

Once you've mastered this way of deep breathing I recommend you do 'energized breathing' three or four times a day so that you are fully oxygenated throughout the day:

- breathe in deeply for a count of four
- hold your breath for sixteen counts
- breathe out for eight counts

- Repeat ten times

WATER

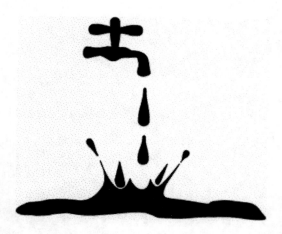

Just like Planet Earth, our bodies are made up of 70% water and 30% mass. This means that the intake into your body should comprise 70% water and water-rich foods.

Drinking lots of water is beneficial for losing excess fat in the body. It also helps in preventing mood swings, premature ageing, fine lines, wrinkles, dark circles under the eyes and high blood pressure, and it keeps the skin more supple.

Most people tend to take in much less than necessary, so what the body does is adjust and hold onto the water it has, which is why so many people are overweight. The body holds onto water to ensure some kind of balance.

Our body cells need plenty of water to stay hydrated and to flush out toxins and poisons. Water cannot be stored in the body, therefore we need to continually replenish supplies.

This means drinking plenty of pure water. Although drinks like tea and coffee contain water they do not count as they contain harmful chemicals and caffeine that actually dehydrate the body.

EAT THE RIGHT FOODS

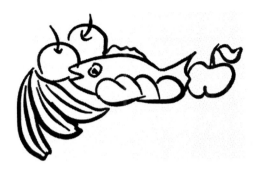

Many people do not realise the link between nutrition and health and energy.

Foods that are water-rich are great for you. Foods in this category include fruit and vegetables. Vegetables are better as they do not contain the sugars that fruit does.

I recently came across the work of Dr Robert Young, the world-renowned nutritionist and microbiologist. He has found that some foods have an alkalizing effect on the body and others have an acidifying effect.

So many people do not realize the link between nutrition and the maintenance of health and energy. So many people are addicted to fast food, sugar, coffee and alcohol and do not realize that they contribute to the catching of infections, colds and more serious diseases in later life. Fifty to sixty years of living an 'acidic lifestyle' takes its toll on the health of cells and can lead to suffering in older age.

I base my eating on a 70:30 ratio of good versus not so good food. You need to be realistic as sometimes it's difficult to eat well, if your job takes you away from home a lot, for example. To stress about this will only create negative emotions in your body and acidity in your system anyway.

The key is to organize and structure your life so that you are feeding your body with the nutrients it needs most of the time. For example, I always carry water and a bag of nuts and raisins with me.

RECOMMENDED FOODS

- Avocados
- Raw fresh juices (vegetables and fruits)
- Raw or lightly steamed vegetables
- Fresh fruits
- Green salads and sprouts
- Nuts (such as almonds, brazil nuts, hazelnuts) and raisins
- Seeds such as cumin, sunflower, pumpkin, sesame, flax
- Beans and peas
- Brown or basmati rice
- Fresh fish such as cod, halibut, salmon, mackerel, tuna and sardines
- Oils such as olive, flaxseed and evening primrose
- Wheatgrass and barleygrass
- Herbal teas such as camomile, ginger, rosehip and green

FOODS TO AVOID

- Alcohol
- Cigarettes and tobacco
- Coffee, caffeine and black tea
- Refined salt and sugar
- Chocolates and sweets
- White flour
- Dairy
- Microwaved foods
- Soft drinks

My recommendation is to eat only vegetables or fruit (whole or juiced) for breakfast and right through to lunchtime.

Just think about the word breakfast. It literally means break-*fast* and if you were to break from fasting you would not start back by eating foods such as fried bacon, eggs, pancakes, muffins, sausages, toast and coffee.

Green vegetables are particularly good for you as they are packed with minerals, vitamins and chlorophyll (the chemical that gives green vegetables their colour). Chlorophyll's role in the plant is to capture the energy from sunlight. So it, quite literally, contains the essence of life. Chlorophyll's molecular structure is almost identical to that of human blood so is perfect body fuel.

I highly recommend spinach and broccoli - juiced or raw – combined with other vegetables for breakfast, as that's how I generally start my day.

Remember, this is fuel for the body for the long term. Look after your cells and they will look after you.

As a result of this way of eating I notice that:

- I have tremendous levels of energy
- I sleep deeply and undisturbed
- I wake up fresh and feeling alive
- I am mentally alert
- my emotions are stable
- my muscles are strong
- I have staying power
- I feel incredible

NOTICE HOW YOU ARE FEELING

It is key to be sensitive to how your body is feeling. This is something I know a lot about from my work as a dancer. I have developed a deep understanding of the way my body feels from moment to moment.

The way I feel most of the time is great. The 5% of times when I don't feel great I straightaway look for what maybe the cause. I'm not used to feeling tension in my body, for example, so if it is present I feel it very acutely. I'm very sensitive to even minor changes in my body and I adjust right away.

I'm constantly aware of how all my major muscle groups feel so if I'm having a stressed day I will automatically stop what I'm doing and move in whatever way I need to in order to regain balance in my body. I can spot whenever even something small has gone wrong because I have developed the ability to know how each part of my body – fingers, ears, eyebrows and so on – should feel at their optimum. When they're slightly off-track I know.

Most people are nowhere near this aware and, furthermore, most people in this country live with pain all the time. Back pain, for example, is a major problem for millions of people. But what so many of them do is live with it. They shut it out of their mind and rationalize that this kind of pain is normal and inevitable. They're used to feeling 60% but it doesn't have to be that way.

You should train yourself so that you are really aware of how your body feels all the time. You can do that by taking dance, yoga or martial arts classes, for example.

Tai Chi is wonderful in this respect. You will learn to be aware of your co-ordination in very subtle ways and will very soon begin to realize what feels right and what feels wrong, through the energy flow that Tai Chi creates. You will become familiar with how you currently move your body in certain ways and you'll learn how to change things for the better.

RHYTHM AND RAPPORT

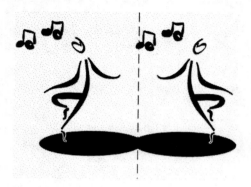

So many people tell me that they can't dance and say it's because they haven't got any rhythm. But if you can click your fingers, that means you've got rhythm and so much of what we do in everyday life has to do with rhythm already. We walk in rhythm, we talk in rhythm, we breathe in rhythm and our hearts beat in rhythm.

The body has great intelligence. All your movements require co-ordination and co-operation from all of your faculties and senses, for example. All you need is an awareness of the sense of rhythm that is already there.

So when it comes to learning to dance, people who say they can't just need to understand that. It's merely a question of linking the fact that you *do* have rhythm with dancing.

It's not a question of either being blessed or not being blessed with rhythm. We all possess rhythm because we're part of Nature. There is a natural rhythm and synchronicity to everything in our world, even to inanimate objects. If you put two pianos in the same room, for example, and play certain notes on one of them, the same notes on the other piano will resonate in line with the first.

When you are dancing with a partner you have to, of course, move in sync with each other but you don't do that by trying to just copy what they're doing. What you need to do is to pick up their rhythm and the steps will follow.

As an example, I've only ever taken one tap dance class in my life and I didn't learn a thing. I learned to tap dance by dancing with other people and simply followed their rhythm. I just picked up on that and found that my feet automatically performed the steps without being told 'shuffle, hop-step, back-tap'.

This is so true in other areas of life as well. You can establish a rapport with someone by tuning into their rhythm and by matching what they do. If you match the way they talk, breathe, walk and even shake hands, you will strike up a very strong rapport with them. You will be able to literally step into their shoes and feel what they feel. You will be in rhythm with them.

Notice your physiology when you feel particular emotions. When you feel courageous, notice how you hold your body. So next time you need to feel courageous but don't, all you'll have to do is to replicate your 'courageous' physiology. Do this with other emotions as well.

ENERGIZE AND STRETCH YOUR BODY

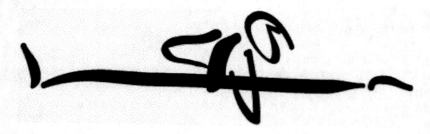

If you're not careful the stresses of modern life will erode your energy. It is very difficult to go after your dream if you do not have the energy you need. If you are holding down a full-time job, by the time you get home and have had something to eat you probably feel done for the day.

People have this impression that energy is something that comes to you. That's not true - energy comes out of you. You create it.

I had a coaching client once who said that his belief was that he had only so much energy available for the day. So he went about his day not doing too much in case he ran out before the end.

In effect, he thought he was powered with rechargeable batteries. The truth is that he could have powered himself from the mains and had an unlimited supply.

But most people try to run on a combination of sugars, caffeine and adrenaline. The answer is to train your body to burn fat (see the exercises later on in this book). This will give you more energy.

Another answer is to surround yourself with the right kind of people. Energy is life. Without energy, you'll achieve nothing. You'll get it from good nutrition and from being in sound physical condition but it is also very important to surround yourself with the right kind of people.

If you do, they will boost your energy levels. Just as the wrong kind of people can drain your energy, the right kind of people can give you a huge lift. You'll get to where you want to get a lot faster with a positive team around you.

Do you realize how much latent energy you've got sitting within you just waiting to be set free? Push and stretch yourself and the energy you didn't know was there will come out.

I heard a great story recently about a top baseball player in the USA. In training and before he goes out to bat in a game, he practises his swing by holding five bats. What this does is to programme his muscles so that when he comes to swing on the plate for real he's able to hit the ball with so much more power.

You too can do so much more than you realize. Just try stretching yourself and see what happens.

DEFINE IT DIFFERENTLY

I've got a question for you – how do you want your body to feel on a daily basis? Define that as a goal.

A mistake that many people make when they think about their physical goals is to think simply in terms of getting their weight down to a certain amount.

What you should do is define your goal in terms of how you will feel when you get to that weight. Think about the things you'll be able to do that you can't do now because of how your body currently is.

Vividly imagine what your life will be like. Visualize it and really identify and relate to the 'new you' that you are seeking to create.

People yo-yo diet all the time because they don't do this. If you identify with how things will be then you will stick to a new, healthy regime.

THE DANCE OF LIFE

The Lord has given me wings so I can fly
I am but a brave and gallant soul
I sense the power that was given to me
I dance my expression to make me whole
- Martin Boothe

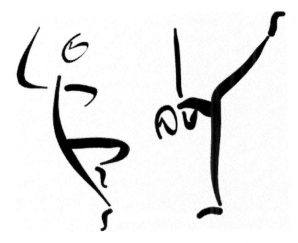

Dancing - what a fascinating way of moving. Life, the planets and the Universe all move harmoniously together. They dance.

How important is dance? If we go back in time, the Testimonies of James Arnold before the Parliamentary Committee for the Abolition of Slavery and Thomas Phillips in 1694 stated:

"In order to keep them [the slaves] in good health it was usual to make them dance. It was the business of the chief mate to make the men dance and the second mate danced the women".

"We often at sea in the evenings would let the slaves come up into the sun to air themselves, and make them

jump and dance for an hour or two to our bagpipes, harp and fiddle, by which exercise to preserve them in health."

Different cultures the world over and throughout history have developed their own unique way of emotional expression through dance.

The Spanish have given us Flamenco dancing, South Americans have given us salsa and tango and Russia has given the world Cossack dancing. These are just a few examples.

All these dances are ways of expressing emotion. Dance is at the heart and soul of every nation and culture. It is the basis of a culture's tradition, social cohesion and ritual observance. Dance is used in many different circumstances such as in preparation for war or sports competition - the New Zealand rugby teams' Haka dance being one such example.

Dance is an art and a form of self-expression.

One of the magical aspects of dance is that it is a positive emotional-state changer. It generates the production within the body of chemicals called endorphins, which create a strong sense of well-being.

Dance is an expression of contentment. It is an instrument of survival. Dance is also a form of autohypnosis plus an expression of love, passion, grief and joy. It awakens our basic sexual instinctive fires.

We have heard many times about how great and powerful men have fallen to the power of sexual, provocative movements performed by female dancers, Middle Eastern belly dancers being one example of this phenomenon.

And yet there are many people who do not dance. They have lost the connection to the creative flow of this vast and amazing Universe. Being disconnected in this way deprives them of the ability to connect to people and things in so many ways.

Through my ability to dance I have become versatile enough to be able to connect to a great number of people. I can relate to so many things - sports, martial arts, movements, hobbies – by appreciating the rhythmic and harmonious way that things and people move.

Bruce Lee is a master that I truly admire and he is one of my role models. He created a style of martial arts called Jeet Kune Do, which translated into English means 'the way of the intercepting fist'.

This means that you do not go against your opponent. Instead you go with their flow. This made his style very flexible as he would adapt to whatever was coming his way.

He gave a brilliant speech where he explained about the flexibility and versatility of water:

> *"Empty your mind. Be formless, shapeless, like water.*
> *When you put water into a cup, it becomes the cup;*
> *When you put water into a bottle, it becomes the bottle;*
> *When you put water into a teapot, it becomes the teapot.*
> *Now water can flow - or it can crash.*
> *Be water, my friend."*

This I relate to in a huge way. I always admire versatility in a person, as it demonstrates their ability to express more of themselves and to connect to so many different things.

As I said before, as a child my idol was the footballer George Best. He was not only a great player, but he was also amazingly versatile. He could play well anywhere on the pitch.

This is a quality I picked up myself. So now I have a diverse set of friends and interests. I love many types of music and have the ability to play many different sports. I am able to participate in many different types of martial art, exercise and dance.

For me all of life is dance, only the choreography varies. It's all self-expression of the body. If you master your co-ordination you become flexible and versatile like water.

Coaching comes quite naturally to me because of dance. Reaching goals and confronting fears are all things I had to do throughout my dancing career. Before I started to dance I was a very shy and quiet person. I didn't express much in the way of emotion.

As a dancer I have since performed on stages all around the world and the one thing that I treasure above all else is the emotional transference that you deliver as a dancer. So many people are moved by either dancing or watching dancing because of the energy it creates and the feelings of joy that are often conveyed as someone dances. The joy and pleasure that comes from the audiences is what I will always treasure. Just watch the likes of Fred Astaire, Gene Kelly, Ginger Rogers, Debbie Allen, The Nicolas Brothers, Michael Jackson etc...

We must dance. We simply must.

A good friend of mine explained to me that when she was going to give birth to her children, she danced around the room. She did this in order to keep in the rhythm of the process of childbirth and to change her emotional state.

When a person cannot move forward through fear it is because of the frozen emotional state they are in. If they change their physiology and experience the right emotional state, then something can be done to improve the situation. The more we are aware of how we feel, the more we can do something about it.

I had a coaching client who felt rejected throughout every aspect of dating. She felt rejected if her dates didn't call her back or cancelled the second date. This led her to feel unattractive and unworthy of being with someone.

We worked together on a few exercises that physically and mentally unleashed her from this rut. She began to appreciate her qualities and grew in confidence.

From that point onwards she went on dates with the attitude of 'if they do not want or cannot appreciate all of this that I've got, then it's their loss'. She eventually found a man that appreciated her qualities, as at last, they were truly out there. She was no longer a shy, retiring person hiding what she possessed.

This is why it is important to dance and move. Learn to salsa or tango. Learn to unleash and connect to this powerful way of moving.

When you physically do something different, rather than just talk about change, results happen. Emotion is motion. Here is an exercise that will enhance your feeling of emotion through the power of dance.

THE 'DANCE OF EMOTION' EXERCISE

First, find a place where you can be totally alone and free to express yourself.

1. Take 3 deep breaths and then think of the emotion you would love to experience - love, passion, happiness, power, joy, courage or whatever.
2. Find some music that will ignite that emotion for you and play it.
3. Then, go back to a time in your life when you experienced this emotion. Put your whole body back there so that you vividly and fully relive the experience.
4. Experience the same feelings you felt back then. Put that experience into your body. Breathe the way you did and put the same tensions in your muscles that you had back then. Stand with the posture you had back then and fully engage in the emotion.
5. Now move. Dance. Feel the rhythm of the music playing. Express the emotion like an artist painting a picture. Become the fluid sculpture. Make it more intense. Listen to the music unleashing this emotion for you. Move your arms, head, torso, hips and your legs with this emotion. Immerse yourself fully in the dance with this emotion. Feel it. Dance it. Feel the emotion rhythmically pulse through your body giving you tingles of sensations of this emotion.
6. As the music ends, stay with the feeling and ask yourself this question: "How can I use this feeling throughout my day to help myself and others?" Then answer the question. Write down all the answers that come to mind.
7. Hear the song in your mind or sing it to yourself throughout the day to bring the positive feelings back.

MOVE YOUR BODY THROUGH EXERCISE

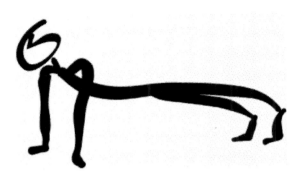

As I discussed earlier, oxygen is essential for life but you need to be careful, as too much or the wrong kind of physical exercise can be harmful to your supplies of it. Such exercise can cause physical stress and can tax the body and result in the build up of lactic acid (the cause of muscle soreness after exercise) which depletes the body's oxygen.

There are exercises that enhance the production of oxygen in the body and they are called aerobic. The word literally means the presence of oxygen.

Aerobic exercise creates pathways in the system to break down fatty acids for the production of adenosine triphosphate, known as ATP, which is the basic fuel the body uses.

Aerobic exercise is low intensity, long duration exercise such as jogging, walking, swimming and cycling done for at least 20 minutes. This causes the body to metabolize fatty acids as the primary source of fuel.

The more often this form of exercise is done, the more the body will tend to use fats for fuel ahead of other sources. This frees up sugars to be available as an energy supply for vital organs such as the heart, the lungs, the liver and the kidneys. The result of this energy supply switching is weight loss for people who want to lose it.

So how do you know when you are exercising aerobically? One way is to exercise wearing a heart rate monitor ensuring your heart rate never rises above your aerobic level.

The formula for working out your aerobic level heart rate is:

- (220 minus your age) x 70%

Another method is the 'talk test'. You'll be exercising aerobically if can still talk comfortably. If it becomes a struggle to talk then you'll have switched into the anaerobic zone and will be taking sugar supplies from your vital organs.

Jogging, walking, cycling can all be done outdoors which is excellent because you get to be in Nature. This allows you to take in all its beauty and this is very beneficial and rejuvenating for the body.

You'll experience the calmness, the smell of the grass, the singing of the birds and the beautiful array of colours that Nature displays. You'll hear the whisper of the dance of leaves in the trees with the wind. This in itself will be energizing to your spirit and will fill your whole being with life.

My dear friend, Master Sifu, who was the European champion at Wu-Shu (a very acrobatic style of Martial Arts), often meditates or does T'ai Chi outdoors to gain the rhythm of the planet.

This is not to say anaerobic exercise doesn't have its place. It does, in relation to strength building exercises necessary for constructing strong bones and muscles.

Flexibility is also very important. You need elasticity in your joints. This minimizes the risk of injuries to bones and muscles through over or incorrect use. Flexibility in muscles also allows for a greater range of motion and freer oxygen flow to the joints. It will keep you looking younger and your skin will be tauter.

Stretching keeps muscles long and lean, which aids the relief of stress and tension. Muscle stretching should be slow and held, as this does not shock the tendons.

Many stretching exercises can be learned from dance, yoga or Pilates classes.

I remember when I first started learning dance that one of my teachers seemed to be so wise for what I thought was his age, that is, 24 or 25 at the most. Then I found out that he was 45! He told me that dancing and stretching had kept him young.

It is important to do exercises that keep you versatile so cross training is great. I recommend you do something aerobic, something that is anaerobic and strength building, like weight training, push-ups, sit-ups and squats, plus flexibility exercises.

Discover exercises that you have fun doing. I find that people I train often do not like going to the gym, so why not try dance, martial arts, yoga, boxing, T'ai chi, kick boxing, aerobics classes and Pilates. Do them all if you can, as variety is the spice of life!

It is important for anyone starting to exercise for the first time to begin slowly. You should not exercise longer than feels comfortable. Our bodies need time to adjust and get accustomed to us moving and exerting them in a new way.

To avoid muscle and joint injury it is key to warm up the body. This allows the body to tune into fat-burning mode and not the quick and short-lived sugar-burning mode. You can then train and exercise in a healthy way.

Your exercise programme should end with a cool down, which brings down the heart rate gradually and carefully. Always wear clothing that allows you to move freely and good, comfortable footwear that supports your feet well.

The most important point to remember is momentum. When you get into a rhythm of moving your body and exercising to aid your health, stick with it.

Before embarking on any kind of exercise programme ensure that your level of health and fitness has been assessed and confirm with your doctor what level of exercise you should start out at.

Here's a two-staged exercise plan that really works.

THE FOUNDATION EXERCISE PROGRAMME

I generally use music when exercising as it stimulates rhythm and helps to make the workout more inspiring and motivating. This is a daily exercise regime I recommend.

1. Lie on the floor (or you can even do this one in bed) and tense and release all your muscles. Start with your toes - point them and then flex your feet back. Do this 10 times. Then move onto your calves and then thighs – make them tense and then release them. Do this with your buttocks, stomach, chest, shoulders, arms, face and then fists.

2. Sit on the floor, bend your knees and bring the soles of your feet together facing each other so that your knees are now apart. Hold your ankles and not your toes. Do 15 repetitions of the 'energized breathing' I mentioned earlier.

3. Then stand up slowly (you may feel light-headed due to the oxygen intake during the energised breathing). Rotate your head in a semi-circle, left and then right, 4 times.

4. Reach your arms up to the ceiling with the palms facing each other. Next raise your shoulders up and down 10 times.

5. With your arms down by your sides, lean your body to the sides, left then right. Allow your arms to slide along your body as you side stretch for 5 seconds each side. Do four repetitions.

6. Then stand up straight and extend one arm out in front of you and the other behind you. Then bring your arms in, then extend them, switching the position of each arm allowing your torso and spine to twist. Do this 10 times (5 on each side).

7. Then with your knees together, clench your buttocks. Keep your back straight and bend and straighten your knees, keeping your heels on the floor and ensuring that your knees stay in line with the feet. Do this 10 times.

8. Then rise up and down on your toes, keeping your legs straight and your buttocks clenched. Do this 10 times.
9. Repeat steps 7 and 8 three times.
10. Then open your legs sideways, a bit more than hip width apart. Keep your back straight and bend and straighten your knees, again ensuring your knees stay in line with your feet. Do this 10 times.
11. Then with straight legs, rise up and down on your toes. Do this 10 times.
12. Repeat steps 10 and 11 three times.

These exercises will strengthen and stretch supporting muscles and will release any energy blocks. They will allow the free flow of energy and oxygenated blood and will activate the lymph system. As more oxygen is fed to your brain, your body will detoxify making you more alert and energized.

Once you've mastered the foundation exercise programme I recommend you move onto this more intensive regime:

THE ENDURANCE AND STRENGTH EXERCISE PROGRAMME

1. Bend your knees and go into a squat position with both your hands flat on the floor in front of you. Keeping your hands on the floor, slowly straighten your legs allowing your hamstring muscles to stretch. Go to where you feel the stretch and hold for 5 seconds. Slowly bend your knees again. Repeat 5 times.
2. Then move your arms in front of you, to the point where you can have straight legs and straight arms. Your body should be in a push up position with your bottom pointing to the ceiling (like a reverse 'V'). In this position - i) bend your arms like a push up and straighten. Do this 10 times. Then ii) keep your arms straight and bend and straighten your knees. Do this 10 times.
3. Repeat step 2 three times.
4. Return to the squat position; come up slowly to the standing up position.
5. Run slowly on the spot for 20 seconds, then run quickly making very small steps for a further 20 seconds. Repeat four times.
6. Then go into what is known as the Standing 8 Counts. 1. Jump down into a squat position with both your hands on the floor slightly in front of you. 2. Supporting your body with your hands, shoot your legs back behind you 3.Go down into a full push up. 4. Push your body back up from push up. 5 Jump your legs out wide to form a 'V'. 6. Close your legs back together to return to the push up position. 7.Return to the squat position. 8. Stand up again. Repeat this 8 times or 12 to 16 when you're at the advanced level.
7. Squat jumps: supporting your body with your hands, the idea is to jump back and forwards, with your legs, over an imaginary line. Do this 10 times (advanced - 20 times).
8. Repeat steps 6 and 7 and then walk around the room for about a minute (advanced - repeat 3 times).
9. Next sit on the floor with bent knees together. Place your right forearm under your knees, then your left forearm

under your knees. Then bring your chest towards your thighs and slowly begin to straighten your legs (as straight as possible) to stretch out. Stay in position for about 30 seconds.

10. Finally lie back. Wait until your breathing rate becomes normal and do 10 'energising breaths' to cool down. Enjoy the feeling of well-being, as the endorphins are released from your brain.

LOOK AFTER YOUR SPIRIT

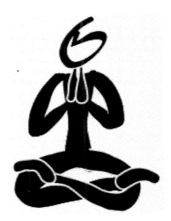

This is the one time I'm telling you not to move your body! I strongly recommend meditation, which is a time to feed the spirit by being free of all movement and conscious thought.

Meditation is the art of stilling the mind. It is a process of releasing everything that's in your mind, and belongs in the sanctuary of the spirit of being. It's a time to let go of all conscious thoughts and your ego. It's a time to release yourself from your fears, responsibilities and vulnerabilities.

We are so busy filling up our time that rarely do we take the time to just be still. Completely still. Yet we must.

Meditation will allow your mind and spirit to become calm, centred, and it will provide you with inner peace. You will then be ready to accept new energy and will have inspiration for the tasks ahead of you.

Meditation gives the mind and body a break from all the activity in the world. When you begin to meditate regularly, you may begin to experience the gap that is the space between thoughts.

It will lead you to internal balance as well as the balance between left and right parts of the brain.

This is really the one time that you will not have to do anything, just be. The key to meditation is to do nothing, not think, not do, only breathe. As thoughts come into your mind, just let them go.

MEDITATION EXERCISE

1. Find a place where you will not be disturbed.
2. Sit comfortably on the floor, legs crossed and back straight (lean against a wall or something solid if you need support).
3. Close your eyes and inhale and exhale through your nose. Take 5 deep breaths counting backwards from 5 to 1.
4. Focus your energy now on breathing and just notice your gentle inhalation and exhalation.
5. Now just allow your mind to empty, as you let thoughts come and go until you have exhausted conscious thought, and let your mind enjoy pure freedom.

This can be done from anywhere from 5 minutes up to 60 minutes depending on how much time you have.

Ideally it is something to practise daily as momentum is key. You get better at it the more you do it.

Meditation is the best gift you can give to your mind as it is a complete and whole transformation for mental and emotional balance.

A FINAL WORD ABOUT GRATITUDE

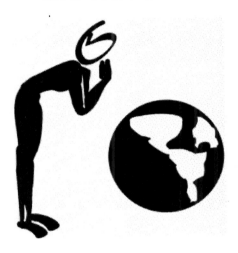

Here's a question for you:

What one thing could you do right now that would make your life better?

Got an answer? Then, why aren't you doing that one thing?

It's a simple question but the answers that people come up with are often quite involved and complex. It doesn't have to be that way.

So let's go back to the question. Think of one *small* thing you could do every day that would improve your life and the lives of people around you. What I'm talking about are the simple things like telling your partner you love them or calling a member of your family to let them know how much they mean to you. What about smiling at a stranger, carrying out a random act of kindness, giving someone a hug and treating yourself to a massage, a sauna, a manicure or a pedicure?

The action you take could be anything - as long as it makes a difference in a positive way and gives you a sense of appreciation for who you are and creates a much more enriching life.

Since I started doing this on an everyday basis my feelings of appreciation have been huge. I am now so grateful for my life. I am thankful for all the riches and abundance that are present in my life in so many different shapes, sizes and forms. Just being able to put a smile on the face of an elderly person gives me so much joy. It is so pleasurable to be able to observe the joy of children playing and learning. I love the fact that I can move and touch the souls and spirits of people through coaching and performing. My life is enriched when I hold deep and profound conversations with people and when I teach and learn more about dance and life in general. I feel that I am truly blessed to have such an array of opportunities to experience the riches and colours of life. Just knowing that there is always more to discover truly excites me.

I remember doing a show in Austria one year just before Christmas. The boss of the agency that I was working for decided to treat his performers to a Christmas dinner. So off we drove out into the country. We parked up and jumped into an air lift and up the side of the mountain we went. Ten minutes later we disembarked to find that our destination was a truly beautiful restaurant built into the side of this mountain! The air lift then left clearing the way for us to witness a beautiful, stunning and truly breathtaking view from our mountainside restaurant. I was in complete awe. I thought to myself at that moment, "If my mother could see where her little son is right now about to have dinner."

This little guy who was once just content to become an electrician and live in his home city was now in another country, speaking another language and discovering a new, exciting life. I couldn't have possibly imagined how it would turn out back then when I started my career.

With life, I'm still like a child always wanting to learn more about everything that I come into contact with. I feel privileged to have this ability to always find something new in whatever I'm doing. I have worked on many shows where I have performed the same part night after night but I've always had the ability to find something new to enjoy and appreciate about it each time. The audiences are always different so the shows are always different.

I love the fact that I can use my physiology in ways that move, entertain, touch and inspire others. I feel privileged to be able to do that.

Plato said that "the unexplored life isn't worth living".

It's all about spending time to feel, learn and appreciate the abundance that life has to offer. Everything and every person has a purpose in life and we all fit in together as one big dance. The trees, the mountains, the animals, music, art, fashion, technology, sport, money, love, rain, literature, food, movies, theatre, conversation and so on are all part of the wonderful mix of life. We live in such an abundant world that we can love, care and cherish.

All of these things can enhance what you feel and, again, the way you move. Just letting all the appreciation of life just flow through your body gives you so much energy to want to move in successful, passionate and joyful ways.

It's a great idea to keep a log of all this appreciation of life in a journal. I keep one and I use it every day to relive and focus on all the great things that happened. I record the small wonders and the lessons I learned during the day. It is also a way for me to feel gratitude and appreciation for the wonders that life offers.

Furthermore, keeping a journal is a great chance to acknowledge and focus on any successful movements and actions that you took that day. We always learn by doing so. Even if you do something that is wrong, as long as you learn from the experience your future actions will be better because of it.

We all say at times, "If I knew then what I know now I would have done things differently." What you did back then was exactly what you needed to do in order to be the wise and aware person that you are now. Your actions today will be the result of what you have learned and earned in the past. Life is never about what happens to us but how we react or respond to what happens.

Never give up on dreams. If you feel your desires in the core of your very being, then they are so right for you. You cannot give up on them. We all have our journeys and we all must move in the direction that is right for us. Doing so enables us to feed our entire being and spirit and leaves the way clearer for the next generation. There is a line in the film Gladiator that goes:

"Some people's lives echo an eternity."

That's how important it is to follow your dreams. You following your dreams could leave a huge impact on the lives of others or the entire world.

We must also appreciate even very small successes in life. We mustn't overlook them as being insignificant in pursuit of bigger successes.

Smile often. Smiling shows the world that your actions reflect happiness, pleasure and joy. It's actually harder work to frown and look sad, so use those 80 facial muscles you've got to create pleasure.

Moving for success is about striving for excellence in all areas of life. Just using your body in successful ways will mean that you are well on the way to achieving excellence in life. Setting and living a great example is the best message to give everyone. Of course this may involve taking risks, but anything great that has been achieved involved taking risks - risks of love, joy, happiness and success.

Be caring and gentle with the planet. This world is home to so much life and to destroy and wreak havoc upon it is selfish, egotistic and ignorant. We benefit so much from Nature and all its wondrous resources. But if we abuse Mother Nature then we will all suffer in the long term.

I want you and those around you to have a fruitful, healthy and successful life by the actions and movements that you take. If you do, then you will enhance your connections and experiences through your emotions and movement. Enjoy the pleasures your body can give and create for you.

Whether it's through dance, song, art, design, conversation or business you should express true, loving emotions by using your physiology in positive ways that will enhance success for you and those around you.

I hope that the information in this book will enable you to take action towards the success you want. To gain more of an experience of what I am sharing, it would be beneficial to attend my workshops. There we explore in more depth the possibilities of movement with emotion.

THE 12-DAY 'MOVE FOR YOUR SUCCESS' ACTION PLAN

Follow this plan to ensure momentum and the building of your success. If you do, you will achieve true awareness of health and love and a sense of vibrancy and vitality in your life.

1. Start to MEDITATE every day for at least 10 minutes.

2. Do ENERGISED BREATHING – do sets of 10, four times a day.

3. Start DRINKING PURE WATER - at least 2 litres a day.

4. Start to eat on the basis of a 70:30 alkaline and acid food ratio - eat lots of fresh greens (raw whenever possible).

5. Create your VISION - focus on it, say it to yourself and feel it in your body at least 3 times a day.

6. Establish your IDENTITY- link your vision to your identity. Find a label. "I am..." - say it and feel it as often as possible.

7. Start to TRAIN AEROBICALLY - run, walk, cycle or swim at least 8 times within the next 12 days.

8. Start doing the FOUNDATION EXERCISES daily. They can also be used as a warm-up for an aerobic workout.

9. Start doing STRENGTH EXERCISES - do them at least 5 times within the next 12 days.

10. Start to DANCE as often as possible. Do it at least 6 times within the next 12 days.

11. Awaken your COURAGE - list and do something new (however small) but courageous every day.

12. Develop GRATITUDE - every evening write down something you were grateful for during the day.

Do this for 12 days. Decide and commit to it and feel the results. Do it so that this way of living becomes your identity. Do it always and live the benefits. Enjoy the experience of moving for success.

I am proud to have witnessed and been a part of a time where people have left such an impact on people's lives and the world. From dance, music, sport, art, politics, technology, spirit and love.

Real heroes. People who have stood strong for what they believed, people that have paved the way for me and others like me.

People that have made it possible for freedom, change, success, love and passion. People that have moved us in ways that have been embedded in our DNA.

Leaders of visions that affect nations, and give them a sense of pride for their achievement.

I honour this life and the privilege to share the same space and time in this world with such greatness, courage, boldness and love.

I am truly thankful and I am blessed.

To keep going takes courage and love.

The two most powerful virtues are courage and love.

I honour you with courage and love.

Martin Boothe

MORE INFORMATION

I'd be honoured to hear about how applying the principles I talk about in this book have had an impact on your life for the better. So please get in touch with your feedback and stories.

You can contact me via my organization, *Move For Success,* for advice and coaching and for the latest information about my workshops and seminars.

Check out www.moveforsuccess.com

Together we can improve and enhance the lives of many on this planet by moving for success in a healthy and balanced way.

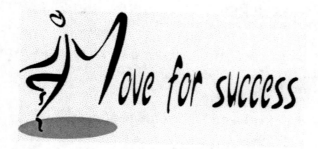